the
DEAN VAUGHN
LEARNING SYSTEM
applied to

MEDICAL
TERMINOLOGY
350
LEARNING GUIDE

DCM/INSTRUCTIONAL SYSTEMS
WESTWOOD, MA. 02090

ISBN 0-914901-06-0

DCM/Catalog number 15028

Printed in the United States of America

This Learning Guide will interact with all previously dated audio-visual program presentations of the Dean Vaughn Learning System Applied to Medical Terminology.

DCM/INSTRUCTIONAL SYSTEMS, a Division of DCM Systems Incorporated   P.O. Box 96   Westwood, MA 02090

CONTENTS

PART I
MEDICAL TERMINOLOGY

PART II
DISEASES AND OPERATIONS OF THE MAJOR BODY SYSTEMS

REFERENCE SECTION AND FINAL TEST

INTRODUCTION

THE DEAN VAUGHN LEARNING SYSTEM

This unique instructional system was developed by Dean Vaughn, who is recognized as the foremost authority in applied memory technology for learning. His instructional systems are used throughout the world in thousands of the finest academic and business institutions with unprecedented success. This proven system of mnemonic instruction and learning has been acclaimed by educators as one of the most significant breakthroughs in education today.

As a student of medical terminology, you are fortunate to have the opportunity to use this organized system of applied memory techniques to learn the subject. It will teach you not only how to learn but also how to remember what you learn.

Countless others have had to learn medical terminology through the conventional method of repetition which is time consuming, tedious, and inefficient. It discourages rather than encourages the learning process. As an active participant in this unique and enjoyable learning experience, you will learn quickly and remember what you learn with ease and self-confidence.

The Dean Vaughn Learning System (The System) is designed to dramatically increase your ability to mentally store, process, and retrieve information. It works in conjunction with the natural learning process of your brain to remember infinitely more of what you see than what you hear or read. Your brain processes images of familiar and real objects faster and much easier than it does abstract information, information that is hard to conceive or understand. The majority of elements and their meanings you must learn to master medical terminology are abstract or unfamiliar. As such, they would be extremely difficult to learn. The Dean Vaughn Learning System converts the abstract information for you into images of real and familiar objects and associates them with the subject in such a way that makes it incredibly easy to learn and remember.

The success of this advanced instructional system is the result of over twenty-five years of continued research, development, testing, and validation.

DESIRE

The most important ingredient to assure your success in this course is your desire to learn medical terminology. Without it, this course will be no more effective than any other. But with the desire, this course will not only be more effective but it will also be the most phenomenal and rewarding academic achievement you may ever experience. In only fourteen classroom hours, you will easily learn what so many others have been unable to learn after hundreds of hours of difficult and frustrating study. Now, prepare yourself for a learning adventure. Be positive, work with The System, and The System will work for you!

THE PURPOSE OF THIS COURSE

The purpose of this course is to teach you the basic design of medical terminology and *how to easily remember* the meanings of 350 Latin and Greek word elements or parts. After successfully completing this course, you will be able to easily interpret and understand more than eleven thousand complex medical terms. This skill and ability will provide you with a powerful foundation of knowledge for the language of medicine.

THE IMPORTANCE OF THE AUDIO-VISUAL PRESENTATION

Each of the fourteen lessons in this course is presented in an audio-visual format. Incorporated into each is the application of the Dean Vaughn Learning System, a proven system of effective memory techniques, to teach you *how to easily remember* the simplified meanings of the 350 elements. The audio narration will guide you through the learning process in each lesson and will provide you with the pronunciations of the elements and the opportunity to practice them.

You will be asked not to take any notes during the presentation. It is essential that you concentrate totally on the lesson presentation and the application of the learning system. Because part of the system's memory technique is based on sound-a-like terminology, it is important that you pronounce the terms along with the narrator as directed. Your success in this course will depend primarily on your ability to remember and recall the sound-a-like terms.

As you participate with the presentation, please bear in mind that the cartoon images and their associations are used to depict illogical, unreal, and in many instances, ridiculous situations. This is done solely for their strong impressionistic values to aid you in mentally retaining and recalling the information. *They are not intended in any way to be insulting, insensitive, or indicative of any real life situation, person, place, or thing.*

THE IMPORTANCE OF THIS LEARNING GUIDE

This Learning Guide interacts closely with each audio-visual lesson presentation. It provides the following functions and exercises required to successfully complete the Dean Vaughn Learning System applied to Medical Terminology:

LESSON REVIEW - reviews the twenty-five medical elements taught in each lesson, their sound-a-like words (audionyms), illogical associations, and meanings.

WORK SHEET EXERCISE - enables you to test yourself on the application of the learning system and the meanings of the twenty-five elements taught in each lesson.

WORD TERMINALS - teaches the meanings of many word endings used in medical terms by relating them to familiar English words.

READING ASSIGNMENT - expands the meanings of the twenty-five elements taught in each lesson. It shows the various forms in which they may be used in medical terms. The reading assignment explains the relationship of the elements with each other and when relevant, their functions, structures, and anatomical locations. Included are examples of each element's use in medical terms.

ELEMENT RECOGNITION EXERCISE - tests your skill in identifying lesson elements within complex medical terms.

After completing the course, this Learning Guide will be a valuable reference for you. Use it routinely to review the system's application and confirm your retention of the 350 elements and their meanings.

THE 100% AWARD FOR EXCELLENCE

This award is presented to those who satisfactorily complete this course and achieve a perfect score of one hundred percent on the final test.* Because this course has been designed for total retention of all the elements taught, it should be your objective to achieve this goal. The award will give evidence of your complete knowledge and understanding of medical terminology as presented in this course and will be a testament of your high academic achievement.

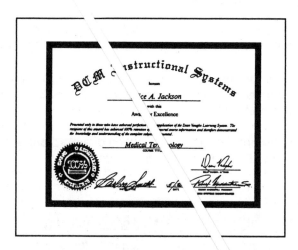

HOW TO ACHIEVE 100% ON YOUR FINAL TEST

1. Pay close attention and carefully participate with the audiovisual presentation of each lesson as directed.

2. During the presentation, be sure to pronounce each element, its sound-a-like word (audionym, as it is called by The System), and its meaning along with the narrator. It is important to pronounce the words aloud. If this is not possible pronounce them in an almost silent whisper.

3. After each lesson presentation, complete the Lesson Review Exercise provided in this Learning Guide. Carefully review each element and picture in your mind its associated image as depicted in the lesson's presentation.

4. After reviewing the lesson, complete its Work Sheet Exercise provided on the following page. Be sure to perform each step of the learning system in recalling the meaning of the element.

5. If you have difficulty in the Work Sheet Exercise recalling the meaning of an element or its associated learning steps, go back and review that element again.

6. After completing all fourteen lesson presentations and their corresponding Learning Guide activities, perform a final review of all 350 elements.

7. Always use these steps to recall a meaning: **Pronounce** the element; **Think** of the audionym; **Picture** the illogical association; **Recall** the meaning.

    (Suggestion: have a friend or fellow student quiz you in your knowledge of the 350 elements before taking the final test)

The use of the Dean Vaughn Learning System is but an initial means for you to quickly remember and effectively apply the 350 elements taught in this course. Eventually, as you become more familiar with them, it will be unnecessary for you to use The System. Do not try to rush the process. Always use The System to recall and confirm the meaning of a word or element within a medical term until the meaning is permanently established in your mind.

* Presented solely at the discretion of the provider of this course to you.

IMPORTANT DEFINITIONS

ELEMENT — a word part used to form a **medical term.** All **elements** in a medical term are essential to its meaning. Each element in a medical term has its own meaning.

Example:

Element	Element	Element	=	Medical Term
nephr	aden	oma		nephradenoma

MEDICAL TERM — a **medical term** is a word or phrase made up of **elements** to express a specific idea

ROOT (ELEMENT) — the main **element** within a **medical term.** Often there is more than one **root element** within the **medical term.** The **root element** is always the subject or main topic of the medical term — frequently a body part.

PREFIX (ELEMENT) — an **element** used at the beginning of a **medical term** which changes in some manner the meaning of the medical term or makes it more specific.

Example:

Prefix	+ Medical Term =	Medical Term w/Prefix	Meaning
hemi (half)	+ gastrectomy =	hemigastrectomy	surgical removal of **half** of the stomach

SUFFIX (ELEMENT) — an element at the end of a medical term (after the root element) which frequently describes a condition of a body part or an action to a body part.

WORD TERMINAL — a word terminal is a suffix or word ending which denotes the part of speech of the medical term (noun, verb, adjective).

Examples of word terminals:

The following word terminals are used in your everyday vocabulary. They will be used in your reading assignments.

Adjective terminals (pertaining to)	Noun terminals
-ic	-y
-al	-ia
-ical	-um
-ac	-is
	-a (ae — plural)

COMBINING VOWEL — a combining vowel (usually **o** or **i** and, less frequently **u**) is used between two elements of a medical term to make the term easier to pronounce. Occasionally the other vowels may be used.

Example:

without combining vowel: hepatmalacia (hepat/malacia)
with combining vowel: hepatomalacia (hepat/o/malacia)

IMPORTANT DEFINITIONS

COMBINING FORM — a combining form is a root with an added combining vowel which the root usually carries when used in combination with another element.

Example:

Root	+	Combining Vowel	+	Another Element
gastr		o		enteric

Medical Term	Meaning
gastroenteric	pertaining to the stomach and intestines

You will notice that we teach certain basic root elements in their combining forms. We have chosen to do so because of their frequent use and familiarity in medical terminology today.

PART I
MEDICAL TERMINOLOGY
Lesson 1 — Review

ELEMENT	AUDIONYM	VISUAL IMAGE	MEANING
gastr-	gas truck	See the **gas tr**uck with a **stomach** for a tank!	stomach
cardi-	card	See the people playing **card**s with real live **heart**s!	heart
megal-	my gal	See **my gal** as the most **enlarged** gal in the world!	enlarged
-itis	I test	See the teacher saying, "**I tes**t" as she stands **in flames**!	inflammation
dermat-	doormat	See the **doormat** made of **skin!**	skin
plast-	plastic (cement)	See the tube of **plast**ic cement with the **surgeon** coming out to **repair** something!	surgical repair, plastic repair
cerebr-	zebra	See the **zebra** with a **brain** for a head!	brain
path-	path	See the **path** with **daisies** growing on it!	disease
-ectomy	exit Tommy	See the **exit Tommy** is **surgically removing**!	surgical removal of all or part of
enter-	enter (sign)	See the **enter** sign made of **intestines**!	intestines (usually small)
-osis	Oh Sis!	See "**Oh Sis!**" holding the air-**condition**er!	condition, any condition
-otomy	Oh Tommy!	See Tommy's mother saying, "**Oh Tommy!** you **cut into** the wall!"!	cut into, incision into

16

Lesson 1 — Review

ELEMENT	AUDIONYM	VISUAL IMAGE	MEANING
aden-	a den	See **a den** with **gland**s growing on the walls!	gland
angi-	angel	See the **ange**l with blood **vessel**s!	vessel (usually blood)
-oma	Oh Ma!	See the children saying, "Oh **Ma!, two more!**"	tumor
nephr-	nephew	See the **neph**ew, the **kid** on the k**nee**!	kidney
hepat-	he pat	See the man as **he pat**s the **liver**!	liver
arthr-	art	See the **art** with **joint**s!	joint
blephar-	blue fur	See the lady wearing a **blue fur** covered with **eyelid**s!	eyelid
-ologist	hollow chest	See the man with the h**ollow chest** for books: He is a **specialist**!	a specialist in the study of
rhin-	rhinoceros	See the **rhin**oceros with a human **nose** growing on it!	nose
gingiv-	gingerbread (man)	See the **ginger**bread man with **gum** stuck to him!	gum
-malacia	my late show (TV)	See the TV set (**my la**te s**h**ow) It is very **soft**!	soft soft condition
-ology	hollow cheese	See the h**ollow che**ese with the people making a **study of** it!	study of
spasm	spaceman	See the **space**man being forced to sign the **involuntary contract**!	involuntary contraction

Lesson 1 — Worksheet

Complete the following:

ELEMENT	AUDIONYM	MEANING
gastr-	_____	_____
cardi-	_____	_____
megal-	_____	_____
-itis	_____	_____
dermat-	_____	_____
plast-	_____	_____
cerebr-	_____	_____
path-	_____	_____
-ectomy	_____	_____
enter-	_____	_____
-osis	_____	_____
-otomy	_____	_____
aden-	_____	_____
angi-	_____	_____
-oma	_____	_____
nephr-	_____	_____
hepat-	_____	_____
arthr-	_____	_____
blephar-	_____	_____
-ologist	_____	_____
rhin-	_____	_____
gingiv-	_____	_____
-malacia	_____	_____
-ology	_____	_____
spasm	_____	_____

Lesson 1 — Word Terminals

-ic, -al, ac   pertaining to

These terminals mean "pertaining to" when attached to a root or a combination of elements. Included under the meaning "pertaining to" are such ideas as:

"of or belonging to or having to do with" (histor/ic)
"of the nature of" (angel/ic, hero/ic)
"connected with" (athlet/ic, artist/ic)

Note: The terminal **-ac** is not as widely used, either in common English or medical words, as are the **-ic, -al, -ical** terminals

Example:
cardiac (cardi/ac) — "connected with the heart"; "of the heart"

-ical   combination of -ic and -al but carries the same meaning "pertaining to" as set forth above under -ic, -al and -ac.

Examples:
mathemat/ical, method/ical, pract/ical, geograph/ical

-y   the act of or result of an action; a condition or quality

Examples:
dreamy (dream/y) — the condition or quality of exhibiting a dreamlike state
inquiry (inquir/y) — the act of or result of asking questions (inquiring)

-ia   a disease; an unhealthy state or condition

This terminal is widely used to name diseases such as dipther/ia, pneumon/ia, leukem/ia.

It may also be used to denote an unhealthy (morbid) condition such as:
amnesia (amnes/ia) — loss of memory
anesthesia (anesthes/ia) — loss of feeling
phobia (phob/ia) — abnormal fear

-um   noun ending; used to form the name of a thing from the root

Examples:
addendum (addend/um) — something added
momentum (moment/um) — something moving; a force

-is   noun ending; used to form the name of a thing from the root

Example:
dermis (derm/is) — the skin

OVERCOMING PROBLEMS OF LITERAL INTERPRETATIONS

Since the majority of medical terms used in the practice of medicine are compound English derivatives of Latin and Greek words or parts of words, it is impossible to always have word for word or part of word translation or similarity in their interpretation.

To be certain that you are accurately interpreting a medical term, it will be necessary at times to refer to an authoritative medical dictionary. Failure to do this may result in an inaccurate interpretation.

Example:
cardiectomy (cardi = heart, ectomy = surgical removal of all or part of); therefore one might reasonably (but inaccurately) assume that cardiectomy means surgical removal of all or part of the heart. To quote one authoritative source, cardiectomy means "surgical removal of the upper end of the stomach or the portion closest to the heart..." Cardiectomized, however, means having the heart surgically removed.

Note: The meaning of this medical term was probably derived from the fact that the upper end of the stomach is the cardiac end or the end toward the end of the heart. In any case, it clearly emphasizes the importance of referring to an authoritative medical dictionary when needed rather than accepting the literal interpretation of a medical term.

Lesson 1 — Reading Assignment

aden-   a gland; a body part that separates certain elements and secretes them in a form for the body to use or for elimination (e.g. sweat, urine)

Examples of glands:

Gland	Secretion
kidney	urine
mammary (mamm = breast)	milk
salivary	saliva

Examples:
    adenic (aden/ic) — pertaining to a gland or the glands
    adenopathy (aden/o/path/y) — any disease of a gland
    adenectomy (aden/ectomy) — surgical removal (excision) of all or part of a gland
    adenosis (aden/osis) — any condition of a gland
    adenotomy (aden/otomy) — cutting into (incision of) a gland
    adenoma (aden/oma) — a tumor with a glandlike structure (a glandular tumor)

Important: **Adenoma** does **not** mean tumor of a gland. An **adenoma is** a tumor with a glandlike structure (a glandular tumor) of any body part.

Examples of adenoma:

blepharadenoma (blephar/aden/oma) — a glandular tumor of the eyelid (an adenoma of the eyelid)

nephradenoma (nephr/aden/oma) — a glandular tumor of the kidney (an adenoma of the kidney)

angi-   This element means "vessel" and therefore may be used to designate any of the tubes, ducts or canals which convey the fluids of the body. However, its principal reference is to a blood vessel or the blood vessels.

Examples:
    angiitis (angi/itis) — inflammation of a vessel or vessels — usually a blood vessel
    angiectomy (angi/ectomy — surgical removal of a vessel or vessels
    angiomegaly (angi/o/megal/y) — enlargement of a vessel or vessels
    angiopathy (angi/o/path/y) — any disease of a vessel or vessels
    angiomalacia (angi/o/malacia) — softening of a vessel or vessels
    angiosis (angi/osis) — any condition of a vessel or vessels

Note: Osis is often used to denote a disease; therefore, angiosis could also mean any disease of the vessels.

arthr-   a joint; a joint of the body; the point where two bones come together

Examples:
    arthral (arthr/al) — pertaining to a joint
    arthritis (arthr/itis) — inflammation of a joint
    arthrotomy (arthr/otomy) — cutting into or incision of a joint
    arthrosis (arthr/osis) — any condition or disease of a joint
    arthropathy (arthr/o/path/y) — any disease of a joint
    arthrectomy (arthr/ectomy) — surgical removal or excision of a joint
    arthroplasty (arthr/o/plast/y) — plastic repair (or surgery) of a joint

blephar-   the eyelid

Lesson 1 — Reading Assignment

Examples:
blepharal (blephar/al) — pertaining to the eyelid
blepharoplasty (blephar/o/plast/y) — plastic repair or surgery of an eyelid
blepharospasm (blephar/o/spasm) — involuntary contractions of the eyelid
blepharadenoma (blephar/aden/oma) — a glandular tumor of the eyelid
blepharitis (blephar/itis) — inflammation of an eyelid
blepharectomy (blephar/ectomy) — surgical removal (excision) of all or part of the eyelid

cardi- the heart

Examples:
cardiac (cardi/ac) — pertaining to the heart
cardiopathy (cardi/o/path/y) — any disease of the heart
carditis (card/itis) — inflammation of the heart
cardiology (cardi/ology) — the study of the heart
cardiologist (cardi/ologist) — a specialist in the study of the heart
cardiomegaly (cardi/o/megal/y) — enlargement of the heart
cardiomalacia (cardi/o/malacia) — softening of the heart
cardiotomy (cardi/otomy) — cutting into (incision) of the heart

cerebr- the brain

Examples:
cerebral (cerebr/al) — pertaining to the brain
cerebrum (cerebr/um) — the main part of the brain
cerebritis (cerebr/itis) — inflammation of the brain
cerebrospinal (cerebr/o/spin/al) — pertaining to the brain and the spinal cord
cerebrosis (cerebr/osis) — any condition or disease of the brain
cerebromalacia (cerebr/o/malacia) — softening of the brain
cerebrology (cerebr/ology) — the study of the brain
cerebropathy (cerebr/o/path/y) — any disease of the brain

dermat- (also derm-) the skin

Examples:
dermal (derm/al) — pertaining to the skin
dermatic (dermat/ic) — pertaining to the skin
dermic (derm/ic) — pertaining to the skin
derma (derm/a) — the skin
dermis (derm/is) — the skin
dermatitis (dermat/itis) — inflammation of the skin
dermatomegaly (dermat/o/megal/y) — enlargement of the skin; a condition in which the skin is larger than is necessary to cover the body so that it hangs in folds
dermatosis (dermat/osis) — any condition or disease of the skin
dermatopathy (dermat/o/path/y) — any disease of the skin
dermatoplasty (dermat/o/plast/y) — plastic repair or surgery on the skin such as skin grafting
dermatology (dermat/ology) — the study of the skin
dermatologist (dermat/ologist) — a specialist in the study of the skin
dermabrasion (derm/abrasion) — a scraping of the skin in order to repair acne scars, blemishes, etc.

-ectomy Surgical removal (excision) of all or part of a body part. This suffix is used frequently in medical terminology and can be applied to almost any body part.

Examples:
adenectomy (aden/ectomy) — surgical removal of a gland

Lesson 1 — Reading Assignment

angiectomy (angi/ectomy) — surgical removal of a vessel
arthrectomy (arthr/ectomy) — surgical removal of a joint
blepharectomy (blephar/ectomy) — surgical removal of an eyelid
enterectomy (enter/ectomy) — surgical removal of the intestines
gastrectomy (gastr/ectomy) — surgical removal of the stomach
nephrectomy (nephr/ectomy) — surgical removal of the kidney

enter-　the intestines; the twenty-foot tube in the abdomen which completes the digestion of food begun in the stomach

Examples:
enteral (enter/al) — pertaining to the intestines
enteric (enter/ic) — pertaining to the intestines
gastroenter- (gastr/o/enter-) — the stomach and intestines
enteritis (enter/itis) — inflammation of the intestines
enterectomy (enter/ectomy) — excision of a part of the intestines
enteropathy (enter/o/path/y) — any disease of the intestines
enteroplasty (enter/o/plast/y) — plastic repair or surgery of the intestines
enteraden- (enter/aden-) — any gland of the intestines
enteradenitis (enter/aden/itis) — inflammation of the glands of the intestines

gastr-　the stomach; the balloon-like organ in the abdomen which begins the digestion of food

Examples:
gastric (gastr/ic) — pertaining to the stomach
gastrointestinal (gastr/o/intestin/al) system — the digestive system; the combination of the stomach and intestines responsible for the digestion of food
gastroenteric (gastr/o/enter/ic) — pertaining to the stomach and intestines; pertaining to the digestive system
gastradenitis (gastr/aden/itis) — inflammation of the glands of the stomach
gastrectomy (gastr/ectomy) — surgical removal of the whole or part of the stomach
partial gastrectomy — excision of a large portion but not all of the stomach
hemigastrectomy (hemi/gastr/ectomy) — excision of one half of the stomach (hemi-half, Lesson 2)

gingiv-　gum; the gums of the mouth; the tissue which forms the collar around each tooth

Examples:
gingival (gingiv/al) — pertaining to the gums
gingiva (gingiv/a) — gum of the mouth
gingivae (gingiv/ae) — gums of the mouth
gingivitis (gingiv/itis) — inflammation of the gums of the mouth
gingivectomy (gingiv/ectomy) — excision of the gums of the mouth
gingivoplasty (gingiv/o/plast/y) — plastic repair or surgery of the gums of the mouth
gingivosis (gingiv/osis) — a condition or disease of the gums of the mouth

hepat-　the liver; the largest gland in the body, weighing about three pounds; secretes bile into the intestine for digestion of fats

Examples:
hepatic (hepat/ic) — pertaining to the liver
hepatitis (hepat/itis) — inflammation of the liver
hepatology (hepat/ology) — the study of the liver
hepatologist (hepat/ologist) — a specialist in the study of the liver
hepatomegaly (hepat/o/megal/y — enlargement of the liver

Lesson 1 — Reading Assignment

hepatonephritis (hepat/o/nephr/itis) — inflammation of the liver and kidney
hepatonephromegaly (hepat/o/nephr/o/megal/y) — enlargement of the liver and kidney
hepatectomy (hepat/ectomy) — excision of part of the liver
hepatomalacia (hepat/o/malacia) — softening of the liver

-itis   inflammation; "inflammation of —"; a suffix indicating a condition, the symptoms of which are pain or discomfort, redness, heat, and swelling. This suffix can be added to practically all body parts. Notice how rapidly your knowledge of medical terminology expands simply by adding this suffix to the elements of Lesson 1.

Examples:
    gastritis (gastr/itis) — inflammation of the stomach
    carditis (card/itis) — inflammation of the heart
    dermatitis (dermat/itis) — inflammation of the skin
    cerebritis (cerebr/itis) — inflammation of the brain (cerebrum)
    enteritis (enter/itis) — inflammation of the intestines
    adenitis (aden/itis) — inflammation of a gland or glands
    angiitis (angi/itis) — inflammation of the vessels
    angitis (ang/itis) — inflammation of the vessels
    nephritis (nephr/itis) — inflammation of the kidney
    hepatitis (hepat/itis) — inflammation of the liver
    blepharitis (blephar/itis) — inflammation of the eyelid
    arthritis (arthr/itis) — inflammation of a joint
    rhinitis (rhin/itis) — inflammation of the nose
    gingivitis (gingiv/itis) — inflammation of the gums of the mouth
    angiocarditis (angi/o/card/itis) — inflammation of the heart and blood vessels
    blepharadenitis (blephar/aden/itis) — inflammation of the glands of the eyelid
    enteradenitis (enter/aden/itis) — inflammation of the glands of the intestines
    enterogastritis (enter/o/gastr/itis) — inflammation of the intestine (small) and the stomach
    enterohepatitis (enter/o/hepat/itis) — inflammation of the intestines and the liver
    gastradenitis (gastr/aden/itis) — inflammation of the glands of the stomach
    gastrohepatitis (gastr/o/hepat/itis) — inflammation of the stomach and liver
    gastroenteritis (gastr/o/enter/itis) — inflammation of the stomach and intestines
    gastronephritis (gastr/o/nephr/itis) — inflammation of the stomach and kidney
    hepatonephritis (hepat/o/nephr/itis) — inflammation of the liver and kidney

-malacia   soft condition, softness, softening. All body parts have a characteristically normal firmness; abnormal lessening of this firmness is denoted by malacia.

A suffix denoting a condition of softness; this is the form in which the term most frequently appears as in:
    adenomalacia (aden/o/malacia) — softening of a gland
    cardiomalacia (cardi/o/malacia) — softening of the heart
    cerebromalacia (cerebr/o/malacia) — softening of the brain (cerebrum)
    hepatomalacia (hepat/o/malacia) — softening of the liver
    nephromalacia (nephr/o/malacia) — softening of the kidney

In structures which are hollow such as vessels or the stomach, softening would be present in the walls of the structure, for example:

    angiomalacia (angi/o/malacia) — softening of the walls of a blood vessel
    gastromalacia (gastr/o/malacia) — softening of the walls of the stomach)

megal-   enlarged, literally "pertaining to largeness," "enlargement of —," but used principally to denote abnormal size. Body parts have a characteristically normal size related to age, sex, body type, etc. Abnormal increases in size are denoted by "megal."

Lesson 1 — Reading Assignment

Examples:

-megaly (megal/y) is the form in which "enlarged" most frequently appears, for example:

    adenomegaly (aden/o/megal/y) — enlargement of a gland
    angiomegaly (angi/o/megal/y) — enlargement of a blood vessel
    cardiomegaly (cardi/o/megal/y) — enlargement of the heart
    cerebromegaly (cerebr/o/megal/y) — enlargement of the brain (cerebrum)
    enteromegaly (enter/o/megal/y) — enlargement of the intestines
    gastromegaly (gastr/o/megal/y) — enlargement of the stomach
    hepatomegaly (hepat/o/megal/y) — enlargement of the liver
    nephromegaly (nephr/o/megal/y) — enlargement of a kidney
    cardiohepatomegaly (cardi/o/hepat/o/megal/y) — enlargement of the heart and liver
    hepatonephromegaly (hepat/o/nephr/o/megal/y) — enlargement of the liver and kidney

megalo- (megal/o) is another form for "enlarged." The format indicating abnormal condition of enlargement is "megalo_____ia." For example:

    megalocardia (megal/o/card/ia) — abnormal enlargement of the heart
    megalogastria (megal/o/gastr/ia) — abnormal enlargement of the stomach
    megalohepatia (megal/o/hepat/ia) — abnormal enlargement of the liver

nephr-   a kidney, the kidneys; the kidneys consist of two bean-shaped glands in the lower back, one on each side of the spinal column. Their function is the filtering of waste materials from the blood and the production and excretion of urine.

Examples:
    nephric (nephr/ic) — pertaining to the kidneys
    nephromegaly (nephr/o/megal/y) — enlargement of a kidney
    nephritis (nephr/itis) — inflammation of a kidney
    nephrosis (nephr/osis) — any condition of a kidney
    nephroma (nephr/oma) — tumor of the kidney
    nephropathy (nephr/o/path/y) — any disease of a kidney
    nephrotomy (nephr/otomy) — surgical cutting into (incision) of a kidney
    nephrectomy (nephr/ectomy) — surgical cutting out (excision) of all or part of a kidney
    nephrology (nephr/ology) — study of the kidneys
    nephrologist (nephr/ologist) — a specialist in the study of the kidneys
    nephradenoma (nephr/aden/oma) — glandular tumor of a kidney
    hepatonephromegaly (hepat/o/nephr/o/megal/y) — enlargement of the liver and kidney

-ologist   a specialist in the study of —; a medical specialist in —; one who has knowledge of or skill in —; an expert —

Examples:
    gastrologist (gastr/ologist) — a specialist in the study of the stomach
    cardiologist (cardi/ologist) — a specialist in the study of the heart
    dermatologist (dermat/ologist) — a specialist in the study of the skin
    enterologist (enter/ologist) — a specialist in the study of the intestines
    nephrologist (nephr/ologist) — a specialist in the study of the kidneys
    hepatologist (hepat/ologist) — a specialist in the study of the liver
    rhinologist (rhin/ologist) — a specialist in the study of the nose
    gastroenterologist (gastr/o/enter/ologist) — a specialist in the study of the stomach and intestines
    pathologist (path/ologist) — a specialist in the study of diseases

Lesson 1 — Reading Assignment

-ology study of; knowledge of; especially "the science of"; a specialized department of medicine; a specialized field of medical practice

This suffix is used widely in medicine to name the field in which a physician may decide to limit his practice, particularly if he has undergone training and examination in the field.

Examples are:
dermatology (dermat/ology) — the branch of medicine dealing with the skin and its disorders
pathology (path/ology) — the branch of medicine that deals with the nature of disease

internal medicine — the branch of medicine that deals with the diagnosis and nonsurgical treatment of disease. Within this branch are specialized fields termed subspecialties.

These include:
cardiology (cardi/ology) — the field of medicine dealing with the heart, its functions and its diseases
nephrology (nephr/ology) — the field of medicine dealing with the kidneys, their functions and their diseases
gastroenterology (gastr/o/enter/ology) — the field of medicine concerned with disorders of the digestive system. This field may be further divided between the specialties of gastrology and enterology

-oma a tumor; a swelling on some part of the body; especially a mass of new tissue growth

Most applications of this suffix have to do with the composition of the tumor, that is, the kind of tissue forming the tumor.

For example:
cerebroma (cerebr/oma) — an abnormal mass of brain tissue
dermatoma (dermat/oma) — an abnormal growth of skin tissue

Or, the term may describe structural features, such as:
adenoma (aden/oma) — a tumor with a glandlike structure
angioma (angi/oma) — a tumor which tends to be made up of blood vessels
blepharadenoma (blephar/aden/oma) — a tumor of the eyelid consisting of glandlike structures; a glandular tumor of the eyelid

Or, the term may indicate the location of the tumor, as in hepatoma (hepat/oma).

As you progress through subsequent lessons and learn the roots for other body materials such as blood, cancers, fat, etc., you will discover many more -oma words.

From this discussion we can conclude that the appearance of the suffix **-oma** can usually be interpreted as:

"a tumor composed of —"
"a tumor consisting of —"
"a tumor arising from —"

-osis condition or disease; most frequently used to indicate an abnormal or diseased condition; sometimes used in words not relating to disease such as in hypnosis.

Examples:
gastrosis (gastr/osis) — a condition of the stomach
dermatosis (dermat/osis) — a condition of the skin

Lesson 1 — Reading Assignment

cerebrosis (cerebr/osis) — a condition of the brain (cerebrum)
enterosis (enter/osis) — a condition of the intestines
adenosis (aden/osis) — a condition of a gland
angiosis (angi/osis) — a condition of a blood vessel
nephrosis (nephr/osis) — a condition of a kidney
hepatosis (hepat/osis) — a condition of the liver
arthrosis (arthr/osis) — a condition of a joint
acidosis (acid/osis) — a condition or disease of acid in the body

-otomy   cutting into (surgical incision); literally "the act or action of cutting into" — usually for the purpose of exploration, drainage, removal of foreign bodies, etc.

Examples:
adenotomy (aden/otomy) — surgical incision of a gland
arthrotomy (arthr/otomy) — surgical incision of a joint
enterotomy (enter/otomy) — surgical incision of the intestines
gastrotomy (gastr/otomy) — surgical incision of the stomach
hepatotomy (hepat/otomy) — surgical incision of the liver
nephrotomy (nephr/otomy) — surgical incision of the kidney

path-   disease; suffering; feeling

Examples:
pathic (path/ic) — pertaining to disease or feeling
pathology (path/ology) — the field of medicine specializing in the study of diseases
pathosis (path/osis) — a condition of disease; -pathy

The -pathy suffix combines with many body parts to denote "any disease of —".

Examples:
adenopathy (aden/o/path/y) — any disease of a gland
angiopathy (angi/o/path/y) — any disease of a blood vessel
arthropathy (arthr/o/path/y) — any disease of a joint
cardiopathy (cardi/o/path/y) — any disease of the heart
cerebropathy (cerebr/o/path/y) — any disease of the brain (cerebrum)
dermopathy (derm/o/path/y) — any disease of the skin
dermatopathy (dermat/o/path/y) — any disease of the skin
enteropathy (enter/o/path/y) — any disease of the intestines
gastropathy (gastr/o/path/y) — any disease of the stomach
hepatopathy (hepat/o/path/y) — any disease of the liver
nephropathy (nephr/o/path/y) — any disease of the kidneys
rhinopathy (rhin/o/path/y) — any disease of the nose

The -pathic suffix combines with all of the roots listed under -pathy with the meaning "pertaining to any disease of —".

plast-   plastic repair; renewal of destroyed, injured or deformed tissue; reforming, reconstruction or restoration of destroyed, injured or deformed body parts

Some examples of plastic repair are:

Correction of congenital (birth) defects such as cleft lip, webbed fingers.
Cosmetic (beautifying) operations such as face lifts, "nose alterations."

-plasty (plast/y) — "surgical repair of —"

Lesson 1 — Reading Assignment

Examples:
   angioplasty (angi/o/plast/y) — plastic repair of a blood vessel
   arthroplasty (arthr/o/plast/y) — plastic repair of a joint
   blepharoplasty (blephar/o/plast/y) — plastic repair of an eyelid
   cardioplasty (cardi/o/plast/y) — plastic repair of the heart
   dermoplasty (derm/o/plast/y) — plastic repair of the skin
   dermatoplasty (dermat/o/plast/y) — plastic repair of the skin
   enteroplasty (enter/o/plast/y) — plastic repair of the intestines
   gastroplasty (gastr/o/plast/y) — plastic repair of the stomach
   gingivoplasty (gingiv/o/plast/y) — plastic repair of the gums
   rhinoplasty (rhin/o/plast/y) — plastic repair of the nose

-plastic (plast/ic) — pertaining to surgical repair

The -plastic suffix combines with all the roots listed under -plasty with the meaning "pertaining to surgical repair."

rhin-   the nose

Examples:
   rhinal (rhin/al) — pertaining to the nose (same as nasal)
   rhinoplasty (rhin/o/plast/y) — plastic repair of the nose; rebuilding, reconstruction of or forming the nose
   rhinitis (rhin/itis) — inflammation of the nose (inflammation of the mucous membrane of the nose)
   rhinology (rhin/ology) — the study of the nose
   rhinologist (rhin/ologist) — specialist in the study of the nose

spasm   involuntary contractions; a sudden, violent, involuntary contraction of a muscle or group of muscles; a sudden but brief constriction of a body passage or opening; a convulsion is a series of severe spasms

Examples:
   Angiospasm (angi/o/spasm) and enterospasm (enter/o/spasm) are examples of body passage spasms.
   Blepharospasm (blephar/o/spasm) is an example of a muscle spasm since it is caused by contraction of the muscle governing movement of the eyelid.

Lesson 1 — Element Recognition Exercise

Separate the elements, connecting vowels, and word terminals of the following medical words by inserting a slash mark (/) between them.

Example: hepatonephromegaly — hepat/o/nephr/o/megal/y

gastrohepatitis

adenopathy

cardiomegaly

enteroplasty

dermatologist

pathosis

cerebromalacia

angiopathology

nephrologist

hepatitis

arthrectomy

blepharospasm

rhinology

gingivosis

angiomegaly

nephromalacia

hepatoma

cerebropathy

gastrectomy

enteromegaly

cardiology

hepatonephromegaly

blepharoplasty

rhinologist

gingivectomy

arthritis

enterogastritis

pathology

dermatoma

cardiomalacia

adenotomy

arthroplasty

angiology

blepharotomy

gastritis

pathologist

adenectomy

gingivitis

nephrotomy

cerebritis

rhinopathy

dermatitis

Lesson 2 — Review

ELEMENT	AUDIONYM	VISUAL IMAGE	MEANING
-algia	algae	See the **algae** on the lake with a window **pane**!	pain, painful condition
crani-	crane	See the **crane** made of a **skull**!	skull
end-	the end	See the **end** of the motion picture with real people **inside** or **within** the screen!	inside, within
hemi-	hemisphere	See the **hemi**sphere in **half**!	half
oid-	void	See the v**oid**ed checks that look **alike**, **resembling** each other!	like, resembling
hyper-	high purr	See the cat **high-pur**ring **above** a **more than normal** number of cats on the church roof!	above, more than normal
cyst-	sister	See the **sis**ter holding a **sack** on her shoulder **filled with fluid**!	sac containing fluid, bladder
chole-	coal	See the **coal** pile!	bile
hypo-	hippo	See the **hippo under**, **beneath** the table!	under, beneath deficient
-scop-	scope	See the tele**scope** with everyone **look**ing at it and **observing** it!	look, observe
hyster-	his stir	See **his stir** saying, "You **turn us**"!	uterus, womb
-ostomy	Oh stop Tommy!	See Tommy's mother saying, "**Oh stop Tommy**!" as he runs away after **creating a new opening** in the wall!	to create an opening

Lesson 2 — Review

ELEMENT	AUDIONYM	VISUAL IMAGE	MEANING
para-	parachute	See the **para**chutes **beside** each other and the **para**chute **beyond**!	beside, beyond
-lysis	license	See the **lic**ense **loosening** and being destroyed!	loosening, destruction, set free
cervic-	serve hic	See the waiter **serv**ing **hic**cups from the bottle with the real **neck**!	neck
chondr-	cone door	See the **con**e with the **door** and a **cart of leaves** coming out!	cartilage
cyan-	sign	See the stop **sign** with the **blue** paint poured on it!	blue
hem(at)-	hem	See the **hem** with **blood** all over it!	blood
ost-	ostrich	See the **ost**rich made of **bone**s!	bone
psycho-	cycle	See the people fighting over the **cycle** saying, **"Mine, Mine!"**	mind
lip-	lip	See the **lip** that is very **fat**!	fat
my-	my eye	See **my** eye with **muscles**!	muscle
lith-	lather	See the **lath**er on the man's face with the **stone**!	stone
ophthalm- opt-	up thumb	See the **up thum**b (thumbs up) with an **eye** on top!	eye
proct-	Procter & Gamble	See the **Proct**er & Gamble container, it has **Ana**cins pouring out of it!	anus

Lesson 2 — Worksheet

Complete the following:

ELEMENT	AUDIONYM	MEANING
-algia		
crani-		
end-		
hemi-		
oid-		
hyper-		
cyst-		
chole-		
hypo-		
-scop-		
hyster-		
-ostomy		
para-		
-lysis		
cervic-		
chondr-		
cyan-		
hem(at)-		
ost-		
psycho-		
lip-		
my-		
lith-		
ophthalm-opt-		
proct-		

Lesson 2 — Word Terminals

-ar   pertaining to; having a connection with

   Example:
     polar (pol/ar) — pertaining to the poles; a polar bear, a polar exploration

   This "pertaining to" suffix is most frequently applied to words ending in **-l** or **-le** and is in the form **-ular**.

   Examples:
     triangle — triang/ular; circle — circ/ular; muscle — musc/ular; single — sing/ular

-ary   pertaining to; having a connection with

   Examples:
     honor/ary, budget/ary, unit/ary

-cle   small; little

   This terminal forms a "diminutive" which is the dictionary term for a word denoting a small version of the thing indicated by the main part of the word.

   Examples:
     a part/i/cle is a "small part."
     an oss/i/cle is "a small bone."

-e   means of; instrument for

   This terminal is usually applied to action roots (verbs) to denote a means by which an action is performed, an instrument for performing the action.

   Example:
     scope (scop/e) — a means of looking or observing; an instrument for looking or observing

     A telescope (tele/scop/e) is an instrument for "looking or observing far away." (The element **tele-** means "distant, far away.") A telephone (tele/phon/e) is an instrument for "distant sound." (The element **phon-** means "sound" and is discussed in Lesson 6.)

-an, -ian   of or belonging to; frequently a person belonging to or associated with

   Examples:
     Europe/an, Ohio/an, Florid/ian

-ide   a terminal used in the naming of chemical compounds

   Examples:
     cyan/ide, brom/ide, chlor/ide

-ist   one who practices; one who does; one who is concerned with

   Examples:
     organ/ist, machin/ist, humor/ist, novel/ist, chem/ist

-ium   noun ending; frequently means place or region, lining or covering tissue

   See the reading assignment under the element **end-** for a specific discussion of the "tissue" meaning.

Lesson 2 — Word Terminals

Examples:
    auditorium (auditor/ium) — a place for hearing
    podium (pod/ium) — a place for standing

-ule   small, little; a diminutive (see **-cle** above)

Examples:
    globule (glob/ule) — a tiny ball or globe
    capsule (caps/ule) — a small case or container
    venule (ven/ule) — a small vein

-ular (ul/ar)   pertaining to (-ar) a small or little (-ul[e]); pertaining to a small version of the thing indicated by the main part of the word

Example:
    valvular (valv/ular) — pertaining to a small valve

Note: in separating and identifying word terminals you may experience some confusion in determining whether the **-ular** terminal is the combination of **-ul** (small) and **-ar** (pertaining to); or whether it has a "pertaining to" only meaning (see **-ar** above). The principal key is whether the main part of the word ends in **-l** or **-le** in which case the terminal has only the "pertaining to" meaning. The context (that is, the way in which the word is or can be used) will also serve to clarify the meaning. For example, it would not make sense to apply a diminutive (small, little) meaning to sing/ular; the idea of a "little single" is meaningless.

Lesson 2 — Reading Assignment

-algia   pain; painful condition; a sensation of hurting, or strong discomfort, in some part of the body caused by an injury, disease or malfunction of some body structure and transmitted through the nervous system

The suffix stem **-algia** can be attached to any part of the body containing nerves to denote the location of pain.

Examples are:
   cerebralgia and cephalalgia (cerebr/algia, cephal/algia) — Note: Although **cerebr** means "brain" and **cephal** means "head," both cerebralgia and cephalalgia are used to denote "headache" — cephalalgia being the more common term
   arthralgia (arthr/algia) — pain in the joint(s)
   myalgia (my/algia) — pain in a muscle; muscle pain
   cardialgia (cardi/algia) — pain in the heart; heart pain
   gastralgia (gastr/algia) — pain in the stomach; stomach pain, stomach ache, "belly ache"

The element **algia** may be further separated into two parts:

Literally (-ia) "condition of" (alg-) "pain," — algia is the most frequent form expressing pain. However, alg- is a root meaning "pain" and can appear in other forms such as **algesi-**, **algo-**, **algeo-**, **algio-**.

   algesi (alges/i) — form most frequently used to denote "sensitivity to pain"
   algesia (alges/ia) — sensitiveness to pain
      hyperalgesia (hyper/alges/ia) — excessive sensitiveness to pain
      hypoalgesia (hypo/algis/ia) — abnormally low sensitivity to pain
   algesic (alges/ic) — pertaining to pain, painful
   algospasm (alg/o/spasm) — painful involuntary contraction; painful cramp
   algiomuscular (algi/o/muscular) — causing painful muscular movements;
      Note: remember myalgia (my/algia) — pain in the muscle

The use of the different forms for **alg-**, that is, algo-, algeo- and algio-, etc., is to avoid confusion with the form for **algae** which is the name for a group of plants including seaweed and many fresh-water plants.

cervic-   the neck or a necklike structure

Examples:
   cervical (cervic/al) — pertaining to the neck or a necklike structure
   cervix (cerv/ix) — name for the neck or a necklike part of the body

This root is widely used in its form cervical and cervix:
   cervical (cervic/al) — used to indicate relationship to a cervix or to the neck. The cervical vertebrae are those bones of the spine which are located in the region of the neck.
   cervix (cerv/ix) — used to name those parts of the large bones of the body where the bone becomes narrow (constricted) behind the knoblike end (head). The narrow part of a tooth at the gumline is also called the cervix or "neck" of the tooth. The name is applied to the narrow (constricted) parts of pearshaped organs such as the uterus and the gall and urinary bladders.

Examples:
   cervicofacial (cervic/o/fac/i/al) — pertaining to the neck and face
   cervicoplasty (cervic/o/plast/y) — plastic surgery on the neck
   cervicitis (cervic/itis) — inflammation of the neck of the uterus (womb)

chole-   bile; gall; yellow-brown or greenish fluid secreted by the liver and stored in the gallbladder (cholecyst)

Lesson 2 — Reading Assignment

The purpose of bile is to help in the digestion of foods, particularly fats. Bile is formed in and secreted from the liver (hepat-) and stored in the gallbladder (cholecyst) from where it is discharged through the bile duct (cholangi-) into the intestines (enter-).

Examples:
   choleic (chole/ic) — pertaining to or derived from the bile; "of the bile"; "from the bile"
   cholangi- (chol/angi-) — the bile vessel; the bile duct, the tube through which bile passes

   Note: Another name for the bile duct (sometimes called "the common bile duct" since it is a duct which is common to [joins] the liver and gallbladder) is ***choledoch-***.

   cholecyst (chole/cyst) — the bile sac; the bile bladder; the gallbladder (gall and bile are synonyms); the storage "bag" for bile (gall) after it is manufactured in the liver and before it is needed by the intestine
   cholangitis (chol/ang/itis) — inflammation of a bile duct (bile vessel)
      From Lesson 1 Reading Assignment: ". . .this element actually means 'vessel' and, therefore, may be used to designate any of the tubes, ducts or canals which convey the fluids of the body."
   cholecystectomy (chole/cyst/ectomy) — surgical removal (excision) of the gallbladder
   cholecystalgia (chole/cyst/algia) — pain in the gallbladder
   cholecystitis (chole/cyst/itis) — inflammation of the gallbladder
   cholecystopathy (chole/cyst/o/path/y) — any disease of the gallbladder
   cholecystogastric (chole/cyst/o/gastr/ic) — pertaining to the gallbladder and stomach
   cholecystenteric (chole/cyst/enter/ic) — pertaining to the gallbladder and intestines

chondr-   cartilage; gristle; a firm elastic tissue serving principally to connect body parts

Important locations of cartilage are in joints, such as between the vertebrae of the spine, in the connections between the ribs and the breastbone (sternum) and in the connections of the ribs with each other.

Examples:
   chondral (chondr/al) — pertaining to cartilage; "of the cartilage"
   chondroma (chondr/oma) — a tumor composed of cartilage
   chondropathology (chondr/o/path/ology) — the study of diseases of the cartilage
   chondrotomy (chondr/otomy) — the surgical cutting of cartilage
   chondritis (chondr/itis) — inflammation of cartilage
   chondrectomy (chondr/ectomy) — surgical excision (removal of) cartilage
   chondrodermatitis (chondr/o/dermat/itis) — inflammation involving both cartilage and skin

crani-   skull; the cranium; the bone structure (skeleton) of the head

Both crani- (the root) and cranium (the name) are used to variously denote three different structures, all of which refer to bones of the head:

1. All the bones of the head
2. All the bones of the head except the lower jaw (the mandible)
3. The brain case or brain enclosure; that is, all the bones surrounding the brain (8 bones). This usage would include all of the bones of the head except the lower jaw and the other bones forming the face, such as the bones of the nose, the cheek bones, the upper jawbone and the bones underlying the roof of the mouth.

Examples:
   cranial (crani/al) — pertaining to the skull or cranium; as a directional term, pertaining to the end or portion of an organ or other body part which is nearer to the head

Lesson 2 — Reading Assignment

cranial bones — only the eight bones which form the brain case, that is, the bones of the head excluding the bones forming the face (the faci/al bones)

craniectomy (crani/ectomy) — excision (surgical removal) of a part of the skull
craniomalacia (crani/o/malacia) — abnormal softening of the skull
craniopathy (crani/o/path/y) — any disease of the skull
craniopuncture (crani/o/puncture) — puncture of the skull to search for cranial disease

cyan-   blue; generally a deep or dark blue

Examples:
cyanic (cyan/ic) — pertaining to the color blue
cyanoderma (cyan/o/derm/a) — a bluish discoloration of the skin

Note: The root **cyan-** also applies to a group of chemical substances. (Cyanide, you may recall, is a poison frequently employed by writers of mystery fiction.) Apart from this chemical designation, most medical terms in which **cyan-** appears have to do with an appearance of blueness (usually abnormal) in a body part, particularly the skin and mucous membranes, usually due to a reduction of the red coloring matter of the blood. The medical words for this condition are cyanosis (cyan/osis) and cyanopathy (cyan/o/path/y).

cyst   sac containing fluid; bladder; a pouch or baglike structure or organ

The spelling "sac" is not a typographical error for "sack." "Sac" is the medical term which is practically identical in meaning with our ordinary meaning of "sack" in the sense of a bag for holding things. The major difference: "sacks" are usually large; "sacs" may be, and usually are, small.

A "bladder" is used in medical terms to denote a sac composed of membrane, usually serving as a receptacle for secretions, principally urine (urinary bladder) and bile or gall (gallbladder or cholecyst-). When "bladder" is used with no other description, it means the urinary bladder.

"Cyst" used as a word ("a cyst") usually means an abnormal sac containing liquid or semisolid materials; a tumor containing the products of inflammation such as pus.

"cyst-" as a word element usually denotes a body structure of saclike form; a bladder.

Examples:
cystalgia (cyst/algia) — pain in the urinary bladder
cholecystalgia (chole/cyst/algia) — pain in the gallbladder
cystospasm (cyst/o/spasm) — spasm of the urinary bladder
endocystitis (end/o/cyst/itis) — inflammation of the membrane lining the urinary bladder

Note: Cyst- may be used to denote both an abnormal sac containing fluid and the normal saclike structures of the body such as the urinary bladder and the gallbladder.

Examples:
cystic (cyst/ic) — pertaining to a cyst; pertaining to the urinary bladder or the gallbladder
cystectomy (cyst/ectomy) — excision of a cyst; excision of the urinary bladder

end-   inside; within; inner (sometimes seen in the form ent-)

This prefix is generally used to indicate (in the sense of "pointing to") the inside of some body part.

It may name the inner lining (usually a membrane) using the form end/o/ _____ /ium.

For example:

> endangium (end/angi/um) — the inner lining of a blood vessel
> endocardium (end/o/cardi/um) — the inner lining membrane of the heart

Or, it may refer to ("pertaining to") the inside of a structure or organ in the form end/o/ _____ /al, such as:

> endarterial (end/arter/i/al) — within an artery
> endocardial (end/o/cardi/al) — situated or occurring within the heart; pertaining to the endocardium (see above)

Or, it may indicate a condition through the forms end/o/ _____ /itis, end/o/ _____ /osis:

> endangiitis (end/angi/itis) — inflammation of the inner lining of a blood vessel (endangium — see above)
> endocarditis (end/o/card/itis) — inflammation of the lining of the heart (endocardium — see above)
> entostosis (ent/ost/osis) — an abnormal bony growth within the hollow interior of a bone

hem(at)-   blood; the fluid that circulates in the heart (cardi-) and blood vessels (hemangi-) carrying nourishment and oxygen to the body cells

Note: You are encountering here two principles or rules which also occur in roots in subsequent lessons:
1. If a root ends with the letter "m," it may also have the form "-mat-." This appears in many common English words:

> syste*m*/syste*mat*ic
> dra*m*(a)/dra*mat*ic
> sche*m*(e)/sche*mat*ic
> sympto*m*/sympto*mat*ic
> trau*m*(a)/trau*mat*ic

Examples of the element **hem-** which ends with the letter "m" being used in the form he**mat**:

> he**mat**ology — the study of the blood
> he**mat**ologist — a specialist in the study of blood
> he**mat**ic — pertaining to the blood
> he**mat**oma — a tumor containing blood

2. If a root begins with the letter "h," it will retain the "h" if it begins a word; however, if the root is proceeded by some other element, the "h" will usually be dropped.

Examples of the letter "h" being ***retained*** when the element **hem-** appears at the beginning of a medical term:

> **hem**angioma — a tumor made up of blood vessels
> **hem**ic — pertaining to the blood
> **hem**atology — the study of the blood

Examples of the letter "h" being ***dropped*** when the element **hem-** appears ***within*** the medical term:

> cyan*em*ia — a bluish condition of the blood
> hyper*em*ia — an excess (more than normal) amount of blood in a body part

Lesson 2 — Reading Assignment

Note: The form "-emia" appears often within medical terms. It means "condition of the blood." Please note that "-emia" is actually "hemia" with the letter "h" dropped.

hemi-   half; half of; relating to or affecting a half or one side; sometimes "a part of"

Examples:
hemialgia (hemi/algia) — pain affecting one side of the body only
hemicrania (hemi/cran/ia) — pain or aching on one side of the head
hemihepatectomy (hemi/hepat/ectomy) — surgical removal of part of the liver
hemisection (hemi/section) — a division into two sections; a cutting in which the part cut is divided into two sections
hemispasm (hemi/spasm) — a spasm affecting one side of the body only

hyper-   above, more than normal; excessive; opposite of hypo- (underneath or deficient)

Although the prefix may be used in the sense of "located above," the sense of the meaning in medical terms is almost always that of "excessive" or "more than normal."

Examples:
hyperalgia (hyper/algia) — excessive pain; excessive sensitivity to pain
hyperemia (hyper/em/ia) — an excess of blood in a body part
hypernormal (hyper/normal) — in excess of that which is normal
hyperpsychosis (hyper/psych/osis) — an exaggeration of mental (mind) activity, especially as exhibited by abnormal rapidity of the flow of thought
hyperostosis (hyper/ost/osis) — excessive formation of bone tissue, especially in the skin
hypertension (hyper/tension) — excessive tension; more than normal blood pressure; "high blood pressure"

hypo-   under; beneath; deficient; less than normal; underneath or below in space; opposite of hyper-

Unlike its opposite **hyper-**, the prefix hypo- carries two senses of "under" in its medical applications. One is the sense of "deficient," "less than normal":

hypoadenia (hypo/aden/ia) — abnormally diminished glandular activity (also hypo/glandular)
hypohepatia (hypo/hepat/ia) — deficient functioning of the liver
hypotension (hypo/tension) — diminished tension; lowered blood pressure; "low blood pressure"

A number of medical words containing **hypo-** carry the sense "underneath or beneath in space":

hypodermic (hypo/derm/ic) — underneath the skin; a hypodermic needle is inserted below the skin
hypogastrium (hypo/gastr/ium) — the region of the lowest part of the abdomen

hyster-   womb; uterus; hollow, muscular organ in the female in which the egg (ovum) is deposited and in which the unborn young is developed and nourished

Examples:
hysteralgia (hyster/algia) — pain in the uterus (womb)
hysterectomy (hyster/ectomy) — surgical removal (excision) of the uterus (womb)
hysterocervicotomy (hyster/o/cervic/otomy) — incision of the neck of the uterus (womb) and the lower part of the uterus to relieve difficult labor
hysterology (hyster/ology) — study of the uterus (womb)

lip-   fat; fatty; fatty tissue

Examples:
    lipoid (lip/oid) — resembling fat; fatlike
    lip- denotes the oily or greasy substance that occurs in many parts of the body:

        lipocardiac (lip/o/cardi/ac) — a fatty heart
        lipemia (lip/em/ia) — abnormal fat in the blood
        lipoarthritis (lip/o/arthr/itis) — inflammation of the fatty tissue of a joint

Many tumors consist of fatty substances (lip/oma), or the tumor may contain other substances in addition to fat:
    fibrolipoma (fibr/o/lip/oma) — a tumor containing fiberlike (threadlike) structure and fat
    myolipoma (my/o/lip/oma) — a tumor made up of muscle and fat elements

lith-   stone; a mass of extremely hard material; a calculus (an abnormal hardening of body substances or chemicals, particularly mineral salts)

Examples:
    lithic (lith/ic) — pertaining to a stone or stones
    -lithia, -lithiasis (-lith/iasis) — the abnormal forming of stony material

    Abnormal formations of stony material may occur throughout the body. Familiar terms may be gallstones (chole/lith-), kidney stones (nephr/o/lith-). The condition -lithia or -lithiasis (also called concretion) may occur, for example, in the joints (arthr/o/lith/iasis), the urinary bladder (cyst/o/lith/iasis) and the appendix (append/ic/ul/ar lith/iasis).

-lysis   loosening; set free; destruction; release; breaking down; decomposition; freeing; dissolving

    lysis may be used as a word meaning destruction; decomposition as of a chemical compound; loosening, as of an organ from adhesions (an abnormal "sticking together" of adjoining parts of the body)

    -lysis most frequently occurs as a suffix meaning:

        dissolving: litholysis (lith/o/lysis) — the dissolving of stones in the bladder, that is, the urinary bladder

        breaking down: hemolysis (hem/o/lysis) — the breaking down and dissolving of red blood cells

Examples:
    gastrolysis (gastr/o/lysis) — the operation of loosening the stomach from adhesions
    autolysis (auto/lysis) — the destruction of body tissues or cells due to internal causes

my-   muscle; body organs consisting of bundles of cells or fibers that can be contracted and expanded to produce bodily movement.

Examples:
    myoma, -myoma (my/oma, -my/oma) — a tumor made up of muscular elements
    angiomyoma (angi/o/my/oma) — a tumor consisting of blood and muscle elements; specifically a tumor consisting of a coil of blood vessels surrounded by a network of muscular fibers

Just as **hem-** occasionally appears in a medical term as **hemat-**, the element **oma-** occasionally appears as **omat-**:

    myomatectomy (my/omat/ectomy) — surgical removal of a muscle tumor (a myoma)

Lesson 2 — Reading Assignment

-oid   like; resembling; having the form or shape of

Used widely in medical terms to name body parts, tissues or fluids by attaching the suffix to other body parts, tissues or fluids which the named thing resembles. Descriptive names for tumors as alternatives to -oma suffixed words include:

   adenoid (aden/oid) tumor — a tumor consisting of glandular or glandlike material; an adenoma
   dermoid (derm/oid) tumor — a tumor containing skinlike elements
   fibroid (fibr/oid) tumor — a tumor containing fiberlike structures; a fibroma

A cystoid (cyst/oid) is like a cyst in being a soft mass but lacks an enclosing capsule which is present in a true cyst.

   lipoid (lip/oid) — like or resembling fat
   myoid (my/oid) — like or resembling a muscle

ophthalm-   the eye or eyes

opt-   seeing; vision; light

Examples:
   ophthalmologist (ophthalm/ologist) — a specialist in the study of the eyes
   ophthalmic (ophthalm/ic) — pertaining to the eye or eyes
   ophthalmolith (ophthalm/o/lith) — a stonelike substance in the eye
   ophthalmalacia (ophthal/malacia) — abnormal softening of the eye; note that the "m" of ophthalm- has been dropped because of the presence of the initial "m" of malacia
   optic, optical (opt/ic, opt/ic/al) — pertaining to the eye; pertaining to vision or sight; by extension, also pertaining to light

   Note: Technically optic is used to refer to (pertain to) the eye and optical to refer to (pertain to) sight.

As you probably know, particularly if you have needed eyeglasses, there are three different names for people dealing with eyeglasses: ophthalmologist, optometrist and optician.

   An **ophthalmologist** (opthalm/ologist) is a physician, a doctor of medicine, specializing in the treatment of diseases of the eye.

   An **optometrist** (opt/o/metr/ist) is a doctor of optometry clinically trained and licensed to treat visual defects with corrective lenses and other methods that do not require license as a physician.

   An **optician** (opt/ic/ian) is one who prepares lenses in accordance with the prescription of the ophthalmologist or the optometrist and supplies eyeglasses.

ost-   bone; bone tissue

This element may appear in the forms ost-, oste-, oss-, ossi-, osse-.

Examples:
   osseous (osse/ous) — of the nature or quality of bone or bone tissue; bony
   osteal (oste/al) — of the nature or quality of bone or bone tissue; bony

   oss-, ossi-, osse- are used mostly in the naming of anatomical parts involving bone and normal biological processes involving bone or bone tissue.

Lesson 2 — Reading Assignment

ost- and oste- are the roots in words dealing with disease conditions and the therapeutic procedures to correct such disease conditions.

osteoma (oste/oma) — a tumor composed of bone tissue
osteopathy (oste/o/path/y) — any disease of the bone; a name for a system of healing which originally relied on manipulation of bones to diagnose and correct disease but which now uses generally accepted physical, medicinal and surgical methods of diagnosis and treatment
osteopath (oste/o/path) — one who practices osteopathy
osteoarthropathy (oste/o/arthr/o/path/y) — any disease of the bones and joints
ossicle (oss/i/cle) — a small bone, particularly the small bones of the ear

-ostomy to create an opening; to provide a new opening; a surgical opening into —; creation of a "mouth"

The suffix stem -ostomy denotes a surgical operation in which an artificial opening is made into an organ or structure (enter/ostomy, gastr/ostomy, chole/cyst/ostomy, arthr/ostomy, etc.) for the purposes of drainage or the discharge of body fluids or waste.

-ostomy is also used to denote the creation of a new opening or passage between two or more functionally related organs:
gastroenterostomy (gastr/o/enter/ostomy) — surgical creation of an artificial passage between the stomach and the intestines
enterocholecystostomy (enter/o/chole/cyst/ostomy) — surgical creation of an artificial passage between the intestine and the gallbladder
hepaticocholangiocholecystenterostomy (hepat/ic/o/chol/angi/o/chole/cyst/enter/ostomy) — surgical creation of an artificial passage between the gallbladder and a liver duct and between the intestine and the gallbladder

Note: The root element in the suffix -ostomy is **stom-** which means "mouth." Since the most prominent of the body openings is the mouth of the face through which we ingest food and through which we speak, the idea of the mouth as a designation for opening was adopted.
stom-, stomat- a mouth; the mouth; a mouthlike opening
stomal, stomatal (stom/al, stomat/al) — pertaining to a mouth; pertaining to the mouth
stoma-, -stoma (stom/a-, -stom/a) — the name for an opening, a mouth, the mouth

Please observe the relationship between **stom-** and **-ostomy** in that "to create a new opening" is to create a mouth or opening.

para- beside; by the side; at the side of; to one side; side by side; beyond
Also, wrong; faulty; disordered

Examples:
paramedical (para/medic/al) — "side by side with medicine"; having some connection or being related to the practice of medicine, such as the paramedical services of physical, occupational and speech therapists. In the last few years the use of a "paramedic" or a "paramedical" has been applied to one who has been trained in limited medical skills to assist physicians, that is one who works "side by side with a physician."
paracystitis (para/cyst/itis) — inflammation of the tissues around the bladder (the urinary bladder)
parosteal (par/oste/al) — "pertaining to the side of the bone"; the outer surface of the membrane covering a bone
paralysis (para/lysis) — "faulty loosening"; the loss, in a part of the body, of the power of movement

proct- "anus"; the last part of the digestive tube, measuring about seven inches in length, through which the solid waste products remaining after digestion are expelled from the body

Lesson 2 — Reading Assignment

Important note: Dean Vaughn Learning Systems has deliberately chosen to use "anus" as the meaning for the element *proct-* in the audiovisual presentation. This was done in order that you might first get a clearer idea of the area of the body to which the element *proct-* applies. We now need to develop the sense in which the element is used to form medical words.

The seven-inch end of the digestive tube (the digestive tube may also be called "the digestive tract," "the alimentary tract" or "the alimentary canal") technically consists of three parts:

1. The *anus* (an/us) — the opening through which solid waste matter (feces) is expelled.
2. The *anal* (an/al) *canal* — approximately one and one-half inches long, through which waste matter is conducted for expulsion through the anus.
3. The *rectum* (rect/um) — approximately five inches long, which serves as a storage pouch for waste material awaiting expulsion.

Technically (that is, in precise anatomical descriptions) the element *proct-* is restricted to words dealing with the rectum (the storage pouch). However, medical usage has broadened the application of the element to include, in many applications, the anus, the anal canal and the rectum in its entirety. For example:

proctology (proct/ology) — branch of medicine dealing with the anus, the anal canal and the rectum

proctologist (proct/ologist) — a physician skilled in proctology

proctoplasty (proct/o/plast/y) — the plastic surgery (surgical repair) of the anus and/or the anal canal and/or the rectum

rectal (rect/al) — pertaining to the rectum; pertaining to the rectum, anal canal and anus

psycho-   mind; mental processes; the processes of thought, judgment and emotion

The element psych- should not be confused with the element cerebr- (Lesson 1). The brain (cerebr-) is a mass of tissue in the cranium (the head, the brain case). Psych- (mind) is used to express the behavior resulting from physical processes taking place in the brain (cerebr-).

psychic (psych/ic) — pertaining to the mind

psyche (psych/e) — the mind

In Lesson 1 we learned the use of -ology and -ologist and applied these suffixes to the body parts of Lesson 1. We can also derive from Lesson 2 such branches of medical knowledge as:

hematology (hemat/ology) — dealing with blood and blood-forming tissues

ophthalmology (ophthalm/ology) — dealing with the eye and its diseases

proctology (proct/ology) — dealing with the anus, the anal canal and the rectum

Similarly, we can derive hematologist, ophthalmologist and proctologist as names for the physicians skilled in these branches.

You might logically conclude that psychology would name the branch of medical knowledge dealing with the mind and that the word psychologist would designate the physician skilled in the mind and its disease. It is true that psychology is a name for "knowledge of the mind" and that a psychologist is a "knower of the mind." There are psychologists who do diagnose and treat mental disorders. Such a practitioner is named "clinical psychologist" ("clinical" deriving from clinic- meaning the direct observation and treatment of patients as distinguished from experimental or laboratory study + -al, "pertaining to"). The field is clinical psychology.

In contrast, the field of medicine dealing with the mind is psychiatry. The root *iatr-* means "healing" and is widely used in medical terms. A psych*iatr*ist is "one who heals the mind."

Lesson 2 — Reading Assignment

To summarize:

An "-ologist" is always a "knower" and may be a physician, "a healer"

An "-iatrist" is always a physician, "a healer"

A "clinical psychologist" may provide treatment for mental disorders but is limited by his license or by the laws and regulations governing medical practice as such laws apply to other than physicians

A "psychiatrist" is "a healer of the mind," a physician and is limited only by the laws and regulations governing physicians

To round out our discussion of "knowledge of," "knowers of" and "healers of" the psyche (mind), you should know that psychoanalysis is a specialized field for investigating mental processes and treating certain mental disorders. Very briefly, the technique assumes that such mental disorders are the result of experiences which have been buried in the mind and that by bringing them into awareness (consciousness) the disorders may be cured or alleviated. You know the meaning of psych- and -lysis. The prefix ana- has a meaning "back or backward." Literally, psychoanalysis means "a state (or condition) of loosening the mind backwards." A psychoanalyst is "one who practices psychoanalysis." A psychoanalyst may or may not be a physician.

-scop-   look; observe; reveal

-scope (-scop/e) — the addition of the ending -e which carries a meaning "instrument for" forms this suffix stem meaning "instrument for observing." The stem appears in words with which you are familiar. For example:

telescope (tele/scop/e) — an instrument for observing distant things (the root tele- means "distant")

microscope (micr/o/scop/e) — an instrument for observing small things (the prefix micr-, which will be discussed in Lesson 9, means "small")

This suffix is much used in the names of medical instruments:

stethoscope (steth/o/scop/e) — literally, "an instrument for observing the chest" (steth- is a root meaning "chest"); a hearing instrument applied to the chest, back and abdomen to listen to the sounds made by the internal organs such as the heart, lungs, etc., in order to determine their conditions

Lesson 2 — Element Recognition Exercise

Separate the elements, connecting vowels, and word terminals of the following medical words by inserting a slash mark (/) between them.

Example: heminephrectomy — hemi/nephr/ectomy

gastralgia	lithocystotomy
craniocerebral	ophthalmomyotomy
endochondral	proctoscopy
hemicraniosis	nephralgia
lipoid	craniotomy
hypercholia	endangiitis
cystolithectomy	hyperadenosis
cholelith	cystectomy
hypohemia	cholecystitis
hysteroscopy	hypoliposis
cystostomy	rhinoscopy
paraproctitis	hysterolysis
angiolysis	parahepatic
cervicoplasty	chondrolysis
chondrodermatitis	cervicitis
cyanosis	hematoma
hematologist	osteolipochondroma
osteoarthropathy	lipoarthritis
psychopathology	lithoscope
lipochondroma	ophthalmomyitis
myoid	proctospasm

Lesson 3 — Review

ELEMENT	AUDIONYM	VISUAL IMAGE	MEANING
cost-	coaster	See the roller **coa**ster with the **rib**s riding in it!	rib
-gram	graham cracker	See the **gra**ham cracker **record**!	record, write
acro-	acrobat	See the **acro**bat using arms and legs (extremities) which are **extrem**ely long!	extremities
rhexis	wrecks	See the **wrecks break**ing and **burst**ing!	break, burst
carcin-	car sign	See the **car sign** made of **can**ned **cer**eal!	cancer
-penia	pen	See the **pen decreas**ing its ink!	decrease
gen-	Genesis	See the Book of **Gen**esis produce an **original production**!	original, production
burso-	purse sew	See the girl with the **purse sew**ing a **sack**!	sac
retr(o)-	retreat	See the men **retr**eating riding **backwards** on horses!	backwards
trip-	trip	See the man preparing for a **trip, rub**bing the car, creating **friction**!	rub, friction
strept-	stripped	See the lady **strip**ping to do the **twist**!	twist
-desis	thesis	See the **thesis affixed** with a **binding** around it!	binding, affixed
mani-	maniac	See the **mani**ac with **Mad** magazine!	madness, mental disturbance

46

Lesson 3 — Review

ELEMENT	AUDIONYM	VISUAL IMAGE	MEANING
glosso-	glossy	See the **gloss**y furniture with **tongue**s sticking out of it!	tongue
-trophy	trophy	See the **trophy** being presented, it is a housing **development**!	development growth
supra-	soup	See the **soup above** and **over** the empty soup bowl!	above, over
-ptosis	toe sis	See "**toe sis**" (the sister with the very big toe) **falling** everywhere she goes!	falling, drooping
dyn-	dinner	See the waiter serving **din**ner through the window**pane**!	pain
mast-	mast	See the **mast** of the ship with a **breast** on it!	breast
-rrhaphy	raffle	See the **raffle** with the suit coming out of it. The suit has **suture**s all over it!	suture, suturing
dent-	dentist	See the **dent**ist with very very long **teeth**!	teeth
cephal-	sieve fall	See the **sieve fall**ing with a **head** in it!	head
auto-	auto	See the **auto** that can drive it**self**!	self
epi-	a pea	See **a pea** with other peas **upon** it and **in addition to** it!	upon, in addition to
hydro-	hydrant	See the **hydr**ant with **water** gushing out of it in all directions!	water

Lesson 3 — Worksheet

Complete the following:

ELEMENT	AUDIONYM	MEANING
cost-		
-gram		
acro-		
-rhexis		
carcin-		
-penia		
gen-		
burso-		
retr(o)-		
trip-		
strept-		
-desis		
mani-		
glosso-		
-trophy		
supra-		
-ptosis		
dyn-		
mast-		
-rrhaphy		
dent-		
cephal-		
auto-		
epi-		
hydro-		

Lesson 3 — Word Terminals

-ate   to perform; to put into action; to bring about

Examples:
intoxicate (intoxic/ate) — to bring about a state of drunkenness or intoxication
fixate (fix/ate) — to fix
vacate (vac/ate) — to make vacant

-ac   affected by, having; frequently, one who is affected by (Note: In Lesson 1 an additional meaning of **-ac** meaning "pertaining to" was presented.)

Example:
maniac (mani/ac) — a wildly or violently insane person

-ad   toward, in the direction of

Examples:
cephalad (cephal/ad) — toward or in the direction of the head
retrad (retr/ad) — toward the back

This terminal is rare in that it also can be used as a prefix with the same meaning:
adnerval (ad/nerval) — toward a nerve
adaxial (ad/axial) — toward an axis

-form   having the same form; shaped like; resembling

Examples:
dentiform (denti/form) — shaped like a tooth
uniform (uni/form) — the element **uni-** means one; therefore, a uniform means "all of one shape"; "all of one form"

-ion   action; condition resulting from action

Examples:
incision (incis/ion) — the act or result of cutting into
action (act/ion) — the result of acting

-ior   roughly meaning "more toward"

This terminal is called a "comparative" by the dictionaries and indicates a higher degree. It corresponds to many common English words ending in **-er.** For example:

Common English -er	-ior	Meaning
high/er	super/ior	more above
inn/er	inter/ior	more toward the inside
out/er	exter/ior	more toward the outside

-or   action; result; that which does something or has some particular function

Examples:
elevator (elevat/or) — that which elevates or raises
flexor (flex/or) — that which flexes or bends
incisor (incis/or) — that which incises or cuts into

Lesson 3 — Word Terminals

-ous   full of; abounding in; having

   Examples:
      fam/ous, danger/ous, poison/ous, joy/ous, nerv/ous, osse/ous

-ure   result of an action; means of an action; device

   Examples:
      exposure (expos/ure) — result of being exposed
      pressure (press/ure) — the result of pressing
      legislature (legislat/ure) — a means or device for legislating, that is, passing laws
      denture (dent/ure) — a device for replacing teeth
      pleasure (pleas/ure) — the result of being pleased

Lesson 3 — Reading Assignment

acro-   extremities; tip; end; a top or peak; extremity of the body; outermost portion

Extremities (singular extremity) is a general word in medical terminology used to designate an outmost or ending portion of an organ or part; a part located away from the center of the body or away from a point of attachment.

"the extremities" in skeletal anatomy (bone parts and structures) technically include the bones of the shoulders and hips, the bones of the wrists and ankles, the bones of the hands and feet. This is the meaning in Gray's Anatomy which is the most widely used text in human anatomy.

Or, the use of "extremity" or "extremities" may refer to:

1. arms and legs, wrists and ankles, feet and hands, or
2. wrists and ankles, feet and hands, or
3. feet and hands, or
4. toes and fingers

Note that whatever the reference, "extremity" or acro- always includes the farthest ends and all parts leading to the farthest end.

Examples:
     acral (acr/al) — pertaining to the extremities or tip; affecting the extremities
     acrodermatitis (acro/dermat/itis) — inflammation of the skin of the hands and feet
     acromegaly (acro/megal/y) — enlargement of the extremities of the skeleton — the fingers, toes, nose and jaws (also megal/acr/ia)
     acrocyanosis (acro/cyan/osis) — blueness of the extremities (fingers, toes, wrists, ankles)

auto-   self / same one; self-caused; occurring within one's own body

Examples:
     autocystoplasty (auto/cyst/o/plast/y) — a plastic operation on the bladder with grafts from the patient's own body
     autohemotherapy (auto/hemo/therap/y) — treatment by injection of the patient's own blood (also auto/infusion)
     autolysis (auto/lysis) — disintegration of tissue due to causes within the patient's own body
     autoplasty (auto/plast/y) — the surgical reconstruction of diseased or injured parts by tissue taken from another part of the patient's own body
     autoscope (auto/scop/e) — an instrument for the examination of one's own organs

burso-   sac; any baglike cavity, especially a sac containing lubricating fluid at places of friction in the body

Examples:
     bursa (burs/a) — the bursa are closed sacs that contain fluid and lie between surfaces that glide over each other. They lie between the skin and prominent bones such as those of the elbows, shoulders, knees, knuckles and heels; they also lie between the tendons and the surfaces on which the tendons glide. They serve to reduce friction at these points.
     bursitis (burs/itis) — inflammation of a bursa
     bursopathy (burso/path/y) — any disease of a bursa
     bursolith (burso/lith) — hard, stonelike deposits in a bursa
     bursotomy (burs/otomy) — surgical incision of a bursa

carcin-   cancer; a malignant (bad, harmful) new growth

Examples:
     carcinous (carcin/ous) — pertaining to cancer; cancerous (also called carcin/omat/ous)

Lesson 3 — Reading Assignment

Cancer is the name used to designate a mass of tissue cells which grow by spreading throughout the body

carcinoma (carcin/oma) — a malignant growth tending to infiltrate the surrounding tissues
carcinosis (carcin/osis) — the spreading of cancer throughout the body
adenocarcinoma (aden/o/carcin/oma) — a carcinous tumor composed of glandlike cells

cephal-   head; the head

Examples:
cephalic (cephal/ic) — pertaining to the head; especially directed toward or situated on or in or near the head
cephalad (cephal/ad) — toward the head end of the body
-cephalus (-cephal/us) — a head abnormality of a specific type

An important use of cephal- is the formation of the combination **encephal-** (en/cephal-). The prefix **en-** has a meaning "within" and is discussed in Lesson 9. Literally, then, encephal- means "within the head." The largest organ within the head is a mass of nerve tissue called the brain. Encephal-, therefore, means "brain."
encephal- (en/cephal-) — brain
encephalic (en/cephal/ic) — pertaining to the brain; lying within the brain cavity

So far we have had five terms which may be creating some confusion in your mind (your psyche) and, therefore, ought to be clarified:

crani-   the framework of bone containing the brain; sometimes used to denote the skull (the entire bony framework of the head)

cephal-   the head in its entirety, including the cranium, the brain, the organs of special sense (eyes, ears, etc.)

cerebr-   in its narrowest application, the **cerebrum**, the main part of the brain in which the higher mental processes take place; sometimes used to denote the entire brain; sometimes used to denote mental processes

encephal-   the entire brain, the tissue structure which constitutes the organ of thought and neural coordination

psych-   the mind; mental processes and activities

To summarize:

crani-, cephal- and **encephal-**   always refer to anatomical (body) parts

cerebr-   mainly refers to anatomical parts; sometimes may be used in words denoting mental processes and activities

psych-   always refers to mental processes and activities, never to anatomical parts

cost-   rib

Examples:
costal (cost/al) — pertaining to a rib; related to or situated near ribs
chondrocostal (chondr/o/cost/al) — of or pertaining to the ribs and rib cartilage
epicostal (epi/cost/al) — situated upon a rib

Lesson 3 — Reading Assignment

costa (cost/a) — a rib
costae (cost/ae) — the ribs (plural of costa)
costicervical (cost/i/cervic/al) — pertaining to or connecting the ribs and neck

dent- teeth; the teeth; tooth

Examples:
dental (dent/al) — pertaining to the teeth
dentist (dent/ist) — one whose profession it is to treat diseases of the teeth and associated tissues and to supply and insert replacements for lost and damaged teeth; also called dental surgeon and doctor of dental surgery (D.D.S.)
denture (dent/ure) — an entire set of natural or artificial teeth; ordinarily used to designate an artificial replacement for the natural teeth
dentiform (dent/i/form) — formed or shaped like a tooth

-desis binding, fixation; surgical union, usually by fusion, that is the formation of a stiff joint through removing intervening tissue and permitting the bony parts to grow together

Example:
arthrodesis (arthr/o/desis) — surgical fusion of a joint

Note: -pexy is more widely used than -desis for surgical fixation

epi- upon, in addition to / on; over; outer (frequently in the sense ''covering'')

This prefix is used extensively to name tissue structures or regions of the body in relation to other body parts.

Examples:
epidermis (epi/derm/is) — ''outer skin''; the outermost layer of skin; also called epiderm
epicyst- (epi/cyst-) — ''over bladder''; the structures above the bladder
epigastrium (epi/gastr/ium) — the upper middle region of the abdomen
epithelium (epi/thel/ium) — the covering of internal and external surfaces of the body, including the lining of vessels and other small cavities (thel- a root having ''tissue'' as one of its meanings; the root will be discussed more fully in Lesson 11)

gen- original; production / originate; produce; formation; bring forth; arise in; be the source of; the beginning of

This is an important root having many applications, not only in medicine but in other sciences and common speech.

The root is an element in many words such as:
gene (gen/e) — the basic producer (generator) of heredity
genit — form for words relating to the reproductive system and the organs of reproduction

genital (genit/al) — pertaining to reproduction or to the organs of reproduction (genit/al/ia — organs of reproduction)
genitoplasty (genit/o/plast/y) — surgical repair on the genital organs

It is in the form of suffix combinations that the root produces (generates) many medical terms:
-gen — that which produces, a producer (generator); that which is produced

carcinogen (carcin/o/gen) — ''cancer producer''; any cancer producing substance
allergen (aller/gen) — ''allergy producer''

Lesson 3 — Reading Assignment

pathogen (path/o/gen) — "disease producer"

Note: Disease producers contained in and transmitted through blood are called bloodborne pathogens. The human immunodeficiency virus (HIV) which attacks the body's immune system causing the disease known as Acquired Immune Deficiency Syndrome (AIDS) and the hepatitis B virus (HBV) which can severely damage the liver are two major bloodborne pathogens.

hydrogen (hydro/gen) — "water producer"; the chemical element
autogen (auto/gen) — "self producer"; produced within the body as opposed to outside sources

-genesis — the process or condition leading to production of

carcinogenesis (carcin/o/genesis) — the production of cancer
hypergenesis (hyper/genesis) — excessive development (excessive production)
autogenesis (auto/genesis) — "self generation" originating within the body

-genic and -genous (-gen/ic, -gen/ous) — producing; originating; giving rise to

endogenous (end/o/gen/ous) — "originating within"; growing from within; originating or developing within the body; arising from causes within the body as opposed to causes outside of the body as, for example, a tissue for grafting which may be taken from the patient's own body (auto/gen/ous)
carcinogenic, carcinogenous (carcin/o/gen/ic, carcin/o/gen/ous) — producing cancer; pertaining to a carcinogen
myogenic (my/o/gen/ic) — giving rise to or forming muscle tissue
myogenous (my/o/gen/ous) — originating in the muscle tissue

glosso-   tongue

Examples:
glossal (gloss/al) — pertaining to the tongue
hypoglossal (hypo/gloss/al) — underneath the tongue
glossorrhaphy (glosso/rrhaphy) — suture of the tongue
glossodynia, glossalgia (glosso/dyn/ia, gloss/algia) — pain in the tongue
glossoscopy (glosso/scop/y) — looking at, observing, examining or inspecting the tongue

-gram   record; write; a record; a writing; a drawing; especially the written record of an instrument

This suffix is used principally in medicine to denote the record which is drawn or written by an instrument. The suffix denoting the instrument is -graph.
cardiogram (cardi/o/gram) — a record made by an instrument (cardi/o/graph) to show the beats of the heart
myogram (my/o/gram) — a record or tracing made by an apparatus (my/o/graph) to record the effects of muscular contraction

radiograph (radi/o/graph/y) — (radi- means "ray" and is more fully discussed in Lesson 8) denotes the act of making records (principally photographs) through the use of rays (principally X-rays)

Note: Although, technically, -gram denotes the record and -graph, the instrument, gradual usage has led to the practice of using -graph as well as -gram in naming the record. This is particularly the case in radiography where radiograph and radiogram may be used interchangeably to designate the record.

hydro-   water / fluid, particularly the accumulation of fluid in a body part

Note: hydro- may also appear as hidr- when referring to a sweat gland and as hygr- when referring to moisture

Lesson 3 — Reading Assignment

Examples:

hydric (hydr/ic) — pertaining to water

hidro — form denoting relationship to sweat or a sweat gland

hidrocystoma (hidro/cyst/oma) — a cyst (pouch, bag) of the sweat gland consisting of retained (that is, "not secreted") sweat

hydrocyst (hydro/cyst) — a cyst (pouch, bag) filled with water

hydremia (hydr/em/ia) — a watery state of the blood

hidrosis (hidr/osis) — any skin disease affecting the sweat glands

hygro — "moist" or denoting relationship to water or fluids

hygric (hygr/ic) — pertaining to moisture or fluids

hygroma (hygr/oma) — a sac, cyst or bursa distended (stretched) with a fluid

mani- madness; mental disturbance / a state of mind in which there is loss of control over emotional, nervous or mental processes

Examples:

mania (mani/a) — a phase of mental disorder in which there is loss of control over emotional, nervous, or mental processes

-mania (-mani/a) — a suffix stem used to signify obsessive preoccupation with something:

kleptomania (klept/o/mani/a) — (klept- means theft or stealing)

megalomania (megal/o/mani/a) — "largeness obsession"; delusion of grandeur; unreasonable conviction of one's own extreme greatness, goodness or power

manic (man/ic) — pertaining to mania; affected with mania

maniac (mani/ac) — one who is affected with mania

manic-depressive psychosis (man/ic, psych/osis) — a psychosis (mind disorder) characterized by emotional instability and striking mood swings

mast- breast / the front part of the chest

Note: There is a small bony projection behind the ear called the mastoid (mast/oid) process, so named because its shape resembles that of a breast; masto- may be encountered in reference to the mastoid process, but usually with a following element which clearly limits the meaning.

"Pertaining to" caution: Words containing **mastic-** do **not** mean "pertaining to the breast" but are related to mastication (the chewing of food).

Apart from the qualifications regarding the mastoid process and mastication, the element **mast-** may denote the front of the chest (male or female) or one or both of the two masses of tissue forming the milk-secreting glands in the female.

Examples:

mastitis (mast/itis)— inflammation of the breast or the milk-secreting gland

mastostomy (mast/ostomy) — incision of the breast to provide an opening for drainage

mastaden (mast/aden) — the milk-secreting gland in the female

mastectomy (mast/ectomy) — the surgical removal of a breast or part of a breast

mamm-, a root applying exclusively to the milk secreting gland, is discussed in Lesson 9.

(o)dyn- pain

This element carries the same meaning as algia which was discussed in Lesson 2.

Examples:

-odynia (-odyn/ia) — state of pain; condition of pain

arthrodynia (arthr/odyn/ia) — arthr/algia; pain in a joint

Lesson 3 — Reading Assignment

myodynia (my/odyn/ia) — my/algia; pain in a muscle
glossodynia (gloss/odyn/ia) — gloss/algia; pain in the tongue
odynolysis (odyn/o/lysis) — "loosening of pain"; relief of pain
acrodynia (acr/odyn/ia) — pain in the extremities

-penia   decrease; deficiency of; less than; less than usual

Examples:
-penic (-pen/ic) — pertaining to a state of deficiency
hematopenia (hemat/o/penia) — deficiency of blood in the body
lipopenia (lip/o/penia) — deficiency of lipids (fatlike chemicals such as acids) in the body
cytopenia (cyt/o/penia) — deficiency of the cellular elements of the body
leukopenia (leuk/o/penia) — reduction in the number of white blood cells; also called leukocytopenia
erythropenia (erythr/o/penia) — deficiency in the number of red blood cells; also called erythrocytopenia
hydropenia (hydro/penia) — deficiency of water in the body

-ptosis   falling; sagging, drooping, a downward displacement

Examples:
ptosis — drooping or sagging of a body part
hepatoptosis (hepat/o/ptosis) — a condition in which the liver is displaced downward from its
   normal position

   Similarly with:

   gastroptosis (gastr/o/ptosis) — downward displacement of the stomach
   cystoptosis (cyst/o/ptosis) — downward displacement of the urinary bladder
   hysteroptosis (hyster/o/ptosis) — downward displacement of the uterus (womb)
   blepharoptosis (blephar/o/ptosis) — drooping of upper eyelid

retr(o)-   backwards / back; situated behind; contrary to the usual or natural course

Examples:
retraction (retr/action) — the act of drawing back
retractor (retr/actor) — an instrument for drawing back the edges of a wound
retrocardiac (retro/cardi/ac) — behind the heart
retronasal (retro/nasal) — behind the nose
retroversion (retro/version) — the tipping of an entire organ backward (vers- is a root meaning
   turning; -vers/ion is the act or action of turning)

-rrhaphy (the word rhaphy used as the ending **-raphy** *)   suture; suturing; the action of joining
together the edges of a rupture, wound, or incision, principally by stitching; the action of repairing
or reattaching body parts which have become torn from or separated from their points of
attachment.

* **-rrh-:** when the combining form of a root is added in front of another root beginning with **rh-**,
   a second **-r** is nearly always inserted forming the combination **-rrh-**.

Examples:
myorrhaphy (my/o/rrhaphy) — a suture or suturing of a muscle
cardiorrhaphy (cardi/o/rrhaphy) — a suture or suturing of the heart or heart muscle
proctorrhaphy (proct/o/rrhaphy) — a suture or suturing of the rectum
nephrorrhaphy (nephr/o/rrhaphy) — the sewing in position of a displaced kidney

56

Lesson 3 — Reading Assignment

rhexis   a word meaning a bursting; a rupture; a forcible tearing apart. Used often as a word ending. Its meaning can range from a bursting or splitting of a major organ to the minor splitting of a fingernail.

Examples:

cardiorrhexis (cardi/o/rrhexis) — rupture of the heart
angiorrhexis (angi/o/rrhexis) — rupture of a blood vessel
hysterorrhexis (hyster/o/rrhexis) — rupture of the uterus
onychorrhexis (onych/o/rrhexis) — splitting and brittleness of the fingernail or toenail

Another form, rhagad-, also has a similar meaning of a split; crack; fissure
rhagades (rhagad/es) --- fissures or cracks in the skin
rhagadiform (rhagad/i/form) --- in the form of fissures; fissured; containing cracks

strept-   twist / twisted

This element is most familiarly used in the expression "strept throat" ("strep throat") as an abbreviation for "streptococcal infection of the throat."

Example:

streptococcus (strept/o/coccus) — name of an infectious microorganism so called because of its twisted form

supra-   above; over / higher than; located or situated on the upper side of; directly above

Examples:

supracerebral (supra/cerebr/al) — over or on the surface of the cerebrum
   (note the limited application to cerebrum, not the brain as a whole)
supracostal (supra/cost/al) — situated above or upon a rib or ribs
suprahepatic (supra/hepat/ic) — situated above the liver

There is a closely related prefix **super-** "the upper part of" or "excessive."

Examples:

supercerebral (super/cerebr/al) — in the upper part of the cerebrum (compare supracerebral above)
superacute (super/acute) — extremely acute
superior (super/ior) — situated above; directed upward; in anatomy, used to designate the upper surface of an organ or other structure or to a structure occupying a higher position
superofrontal (super/o/front/al) — situated at the upper and frontal part of a structure
superolateral (super/o/later/al) — above and at the side (later- which is discussed in Lesson 9 means "side")
superfunction (super/function) — excessive activity of an organ such as a gland; hyperfunctioning

trip-   rub; friction

Examples:

tripsis (trip/sis) — the act of rubbing, massaging
-tripsy (tripsy) — crushing; — tripsy is derived from the Greek element trip-
lithotripsy (lith/o/trips/y) — crushing of a calculus (stone) within the bladder
hepaticolithotripsy (hepat/ic/o/lith/o/trips/y) — the operation of crushing a stone in a liver (hepat/ic) duct

cholecystolithotripsy (chole/cyst/o/lith/o/trips/y) — the crushing of gallstones (cholelith) in the gallbladder (cholecyst)

-trophy   development, growth; nutrition, nourishment

Examples:
   trophic (troph/ic) — pertaining to nutrition, development, growth
   trophopathy (troph/o/path/y) — any disease due to faulty nutrition
   trophotherapy (troph/o/therap/y) — treatment of disease by nourishment (diet) measures

There are some important combinations frequently appearing at the ends of medical words or phrases:
   hypertrophy (hyper/trophy) — "over development"; the overgrowth of an organ or part
   atrophy (a/trophy) — "not growth"; a wasting away or decrease in the size of cell, tissue, organ or body part (a- has a meaning "not," "without")
   dystrophy (dys/trophy) — "bad development"; a disorder arising from defective or faulty nutrition (dys- means "bad" and is discussed more fully in Lesson 9)

Lesson 3 — Element Recognition Exercise

Separate the elements, connecting vowels, and word terminals of the following medical words by inserting a slash mark (/) between them.

Example: hydrocholecystitis — hydro/chole/cyst/itis

costochondral

cholecystogram

acropathology

angiorrhexis

carcinogenesis

hydropenia

pathogen

bursolith

retrocervical

lithotripsy

arthrodesis

glossoplasty

autotrophy

supracerebral

blepharoptosis

myodynia

mastadenitis

glossorrhaphy

dentoid

cephalogenesis

autocystoplasty

epicystitis

hydrohepatosis

angiogram

acromegaly

cardiorrhexis

carcinoma

hypogenesis

bursopathy

retrocardiac

cephalopathy

autology

epidermis

hydrology

mania

glossalgia

trophology

supracostal

gastroptosis

cervicodynia

mastocarcinoma

myorrhaphy

Lesson 4 — Review

ELEMENT	AUDIONYM	VISUAL IMAGE	MEANING
lobo-	low bow	See the **low bow** made of **section**s!	section
-emesis	Hey Mrs.!	See the bellhop saying, **"Hey Mrs.!"** as she is **vomiting** in the lobby!	vomiting
contra-	contractor	See the **contra**ctor leaning the tools **against** the **counter**!	against, counter
-iasis	oasis	See the **oasis** with air-**conditioner**s on it!	condition, formation of, presence of
trans-	trains	See the **trains** going **through a cross**!	through, across, beyond
brady-	braid	See the girl's hair being **braid**ed so **slow**ly she grows old!	slow
-ectasis	"egged a sis"	See the boy who **"egged a sis"** with an **"X" pan**!	expansion
cyt-	sight	See the **sight** of the gun barrel made of a **cell**!	cell
odont-	Oh don't	See the person saying **"Oh don't** hit me with that **tooth"**!	tooth
leuk-	look (magazine)	See the **Look** magazine that is all **white**!	white
-esthesia	has the show	See the man who h**as the sh**ow (holding the stage). He is **sensational**!	sensation, feeling
cantho-	can throw	See the **can** being **thr**own at the **angle at the end of the eyelid**!	angle at the end of the eyelid

Lesson 4 — Review

ELEMENT	AUDIONYM	VISUAL IMAGE	MEANING
steno	steno-grapher	See the **steno**grapher typing a **narrow contract**!	narrow, contracted
cheil-	cow	See the **cow** with the human **lip**s!	lip
-cele	seal	See the **seal** on **her** k**nee**!	hernia, tumor or swelling
benign	bee "9"	See the **bee** stinging the **"9"** which **mel**ts into a k**not** and falls into a **can**!	mild, not cancerous
semen	seaman	See the **seaman** with the **seed**s in his hat!	seed
celio-	ceiling dome	See the **ceili**ng d**ome** with an **ap**ple **dome** hanging from it!	abdomen
erythro-	wreath throw	See the **wreath** being **throw**n. It is **red**!	red
vaso-	vase	See the **vas**e with **vessel**s on it!	vessel
melan-	melon	See the **melon** that is **black** inside!	black
cauda-	cod liver oil	See the **cod** li**ver** oil with a **tail** sticking out of it!	tail
lingua-	language	See the man who speaks many **lan-gua**ges because he has many **tongue**s!	tongue
myring-	my ring	See **"my ring"** with an **ear** and a **drum** on it!	eardrum
spondyl-	spun doll	See the **spun doll** (a doll spinning) so fast that you can see the **spinal column**!	spinal column or vertebra

Lesson 4 — Worksheet

Complete the following:

ELEMENT	AUDIONYM	MEANING
lobo-		
-emesis		
contra-		
-iasis		
trans-		
brady-		
-ectasis		
cyt-		
odont-		
leuk-		
-esthesia		
cantho-		
steno-		
cheil-		
-cele		
benign		
semen		
celio-		
erythro-		
vaso-		
melan-		
cauda-		
lingua-		
myring-		
spondyl-		

Lesson 4 — Word Terminals

-a   noun ending; used to form the name of a thing from a root

Examples:
   derma (derm/a) — the skin
   gingiva (gingiv/a) — the gum
   costa (cost/a) — a rib

Also, the terminal to form the plural of words ending in **-on** and **-um.**

Examples:
   bacteri/um — bacteri/a; dat/um — dat/a; criteri/on — criteri/a; phenomen/on — phenomen/a

-ae   plural ending for words ending in **-a**

Examples:
   gingiv/a — gingiv/ae; cost/a — cost/ae; burs/a — burs/ae

-ant   pertaining to; having the characteristics of

Examples:
   pleasant (pleas/ant) — having the characteristics of pleasing
   malignant (malign/ant) — having the characteristics of badness

-ation   a process, action, or condition

This terminal is a combination of **-ate** (to put into action) and **-ion** (condition resulting from an action).

Examples:
   starv/ation, observ/ation, discolor/ation, decor/ation

-esis   condition or process

Examples:
   genesis (gen/esis) — the process of producing or originating
   uresis (ur/esis) — the process of passing urine (the element **ur-** means "urine")

Note: The terminal **-esis** is closely related to the element **-osis** (Lesson 1).

-ics   the body of facts, knowledge, matters, etc., pertaining to a subject and hence a science or art; the study of

Examples:
   polit/ics, mathemat/ics, electron/ics, opt/ics, athlet/ics, econom/ics

Note: **-ics** carries a meaning identical with **-ology**. However, there is a subtle distinction in medicine. When **-ics** and **-ology** are used to denote a body of medical knowledge, the **-ology** ending is used for the field covered by the doctor of medicine or osteopathy; the **-ics** is limited to the non-M.D. or D.O. field. To illustrate:

   anesthesiology is the broad field covered by the doctor; anesthetics is the field covered by the non-doctor, usually a technician

   ophthalmology is the field covered by the doctor; optics is the field covered by the non-doctor.

Lesson 4 — Word Terminals

-in organic compounds such as carbohydrates and protein

Example:
melanin (melan/in) — an organic compound providing a dark color to skin and hair

-ly in a manner, in a way, by way of, toward

Examples:
slowly (slow/ly) — in a slow manner
smilingly (smiling/ly) — in a smiling way
lingually (lingual/ly) — toward the tongue, by way of the tongue

-tic pertaining to

This terminal is especially used to give a "pertaining to" meaning to words ending in **-sis**.

Examples:
eme/sis — eme/tic; analy/sis — analy/tic; diagno/sis — diagnos/tic; hypno/sis — hypno/tic

Lesson 4 — Reading Assignment

benign   mild; not cancerous / not recurrent; favorable for recovery

This word is used in phrases to describe the relative severity of a disease, for example:

mild vs. severe as in "a benign psychosis"
not threatening life or health as in "a benign malaria"
having a good prognosis (a forecast as to the probable result of an attack of disease; the prospect as to recovery from a disease) as in "a benign psychosis"

The principal use of the word is to designate the absence of cancerous tumors as in "a benign tumor" versus "a carcin/oma."

brady-   slow / slowness; abnormal slowness in physical or mental process

This root is descriptive and can practically always be interpreted as "slowness of" or "abnormal slowness of."

Examples:

bradycardia (brady/card/ia) — abnormal slowness of the heartbeat (usually less than 60 beats per minute)
myobradia (my/o/brad/ia) — a slow, sluggish reaction of muscle to electrical stimulation

An interesting illustration of the use of roots to describe different causes for similar symptoms is the symptom "abnormal slowness of speech":

bradyglossia (brady/glossia) — abnormal slowness of utterance (the vocal forming of sounds to express speech)
bradylogia (brady/log/ia) — abnormal slowness of speech due to slowness of thinking as in a mental disorder

Note that difficulty in physically forming words is conveyed by the use of gloss- (tongue), the principal organ used in the forming of speech sounds. On the other hand, the use of log- (-ology, "study of") carries the idea of a mental process. (The application of the element log- for the mental process makes more sense when we know that the original meaning of log- was "discourse" or "speaking on." An -ologist, a "student of" a subject, had the ability to "speak on" the subject.)

cantho-   angle at the end of the eyelid; one of the corners of the eye; either of the angles formed by the meeting of the upper and lower eyelids

Examples:
canthal (canth/al) — pertaining to a corner of the eye
canthus (canth/us) — name of the corner of the eye

As you might expect, the tissue forming the corner of the eye may become inflamed, incised, excised, repaired, or loosened. Can you form the appropriate medical words?

cauda-   tail / tail part of the body; the "rear end"; a tail-like appendage (something hanging upon a main structure; the "appendix" is a small pouch or sac "hanging on" to a section of the intestines)

Examples:
caudal (caud/al) — pertaining to the tail (the "rear end") or a tail-like appendage; pertaining to the lower and/or rear end
cauda (caud/a) — name for a tail-like appendage

Lesson 4 — Reading Assignment

This root is used principally to indicate a direction, a position toward the tail ("rear end") of the body or a body part. It may also be used to name a tail-like appendage.

Examples:
  caudad (caud/ad) — directed toward a cauda or tail; opposite to cephal/ad
  caudalward (caud/al/ward) — toward the caudal, tail or back end
  caudal anesthesia (caud/al an/esthesia) — loss of sensation produced by an injection of an anesthetic into the lower (caudal) portion of the spinal cord

-cele   hernia, tumor or swelling / an external projection of a part from its natural cavity

In Lesson 3 we learned that the suffix -rhexis named a condition of breaking, bursting, rupturing. The physical evidence of such a rupturing or breaking out is a hernia, frequently a balloon-like protrusion of an organ through its containing wall. -Cele is the suffix used to denote a hernia.

Examples:
  myocele (my/o/cele) — a muscle hernia; a muscle protrusion
  cystocele (cyst/o/cele) — protrusion of the bladder through the vaginal wall
  cephalocele (cephal/o/cele) — protrusion of part of the cranial contents
  hydrocele (hydr/o/cele) — collection of fluid in a swelling; especially in male genital parts

celio-   abdomen; any large cavity of the body, especially the abdomen

Examples:
  celiac (celi/ac) — pertaining to the abdomen
  celiorrhaphy (celio/rrhaphy) — suture of the abdominal wall
  celitis (cel/itis) — any inflammation of the abdomen
  celiotomy (celio/tomy) — surgical incision into the abdominal cavity

cheil-   lip / the lips of the face; infrequently used to denote an edge or brim

Examples:
  cheilocarcinoma (cheil/o/carcin/oma) — cancer of the lip
  cheilorrhaphy (cheil/o/rrhaphy) — suturing of the lips

Other words which you should recognize are:
  cheiloplasty (cheil/o/plast/y)
  cheilosis (cheil/osis)

contra-   against; counter / in opposition to; a thing opposite or against another

This prefix may be attached to a word or stem with the meaning "opposite to" or "against."

Examples:
  contraction (contr/action) — "acting against"; a shortening; for example, a muscle contraction
  contraception (contra/ception) — "acting against conception"; the prevention of pregnancy
  contrastimulant (contra/stimulant) — "against stimulation"; a medicine or action applied to overcome or alleviate stimulation

Counter- which has the same meaning of "against" or "opposite to" is used frequently to indicate "a direction opposite to." For example:
  counteropening (counter/opening) (also counter/incision) — a second incision made opposite to another, as in an abscess, to promote drainage
  counterirritation (counter/irritation) — an irritation which is supposed to relieve some other irritation

Lesson 4 — Reading Assignment

cyt-   cell / a small, usually microscopic mass of sticky fluid contained in a membranous sac

This root is widely used in medicine since it means "cell." Cells are the building blocks of the body. All body parts consist of tissues which are made up of cells. Cells of one tissue differ from those of other tissues depending on the function they perform.

Examples:
   hemocyte or hemacyte (hem/o/cyt/e, hema/cyt/e) — a blood cell; blood cells are of two kinds:

   leukocyte (leuk/o/cyt/e) — white blood cell
   erythrocyte (erythr/o/cyt/e) — red blood cell

   myocyte (my/o/cyt/e) — a cell of the muscular tissue
   -cytic (-cyt/ic) — pertaining to cells
   cytogenesis (cyt/o/gen/esis) — the production and development of cells

-ectasis   expansion / "a stretching out"; enlargement

This suffix denotes an enlargement (in a limited sense, a -megaly) by stretching; the condition of being stretched beyond normal dimensions (ec- a variation of ex- meaning "out" + tasis "stretching").

Examples:
   angiectasis (angi/ectasis) — beyond normal stretching of a blood vessel
   nephrectasis (nephr/ectasis) — stretching (distention) of the kidney

Another way of expressing "ectasis" is the word dilatation." You probably know that dilate means "to expand," "to stretch." In medical terms dilatation means "the condition of being dilated or stretched beyond normal dimensions."

-emesis   vomiting / a condition or occurrence ("happening") of vomiting

Our clue here is the ending **-sis** meaning "condition." Therefore, this must mean a condition of "eme-." Since we learned that -emesis means "vomiting," the "eme" must mean "vomit" and so it does. Eme- is a root meaning "vomit." -Emesis is used as a suffix combination or as a word.

Examples:
   emesis (eme/sis) — the act of vomiting
   emetic (eme/tic) — that which causes vomiting such as a drug
   hematemesis (hemat/eme/sis) — the vomiting of blood
   cholemesis (chol/eme/sis) — the vomiting of bile or gall

erythro-   red / the color red

Examples:
   erythra (erythr/a) — an eruption (breaking out) of the skin marked by redness of the skin and/or swelling
   erythralgia (erythr/algia) — a condition marked by pain and redness of the skin
   erythrocyt- (erythr/o/cyt-) — meaning "red cell," actually "red blood cell," is a frequent combination in medical terms:

   erythrocytopenia (erythr/o/cyt/o/penia) — deficiency of the number of red blood cells; frequently shortened to erythropenia
   erythrocythemia (erythr/o/cyt/hem/ia) — a condition of increase of the number of red blood cells; also erythrocytosis

Lesson 4 — Reading Assignment

-esthesia   sensation, feeling / perception; physical sensitivity; consciousness

Examples:
   -esthetic (-esthet/ic) — pertaining to feeling
   -esthesia (-esthes/ia) — the condition of feeling; a "feeling of"; awareness of feeling
   anesthes- (an/esthes-) — lack of feeling (an- "lack of" covered in Lesson 10)

This root, in medical terms, deals primarily with physical sensations, particularly the sense of pain and the general feeling of the senses (consciousness, perception). An important derivative of esthes- is its opposite **an/esthes-** "lack of feeling" or absence of feeling.

Examples:
   optesthesia (opt/esthesia) — the ability to see; the ability to perceive visual stimuli
   anesthesiology (an/esthesi/ology) — the branch of medical science dealing with the bringing about the loss of sensation, principally as an adjunct to pain-causing therapeutic procedures such as surgery

-iasis   condition; formation of; presence of / state of (almost always relating to disease or abnormality)

This suffix is widely used in medicine to denote a disease process or the condition resulting from disease, literally "illness condition" or "sick condition." In Lesson 1 you learned that the word ending **-ia** means disease.

Examples:
   lithiasis (lith/iasis) — a condition characterized by the formation of stones
   elephantiasis (elephant/iasis) — a condition characterized by enlargement of the parts affected and thickening and discoloration of the skin covering these parts

leuk-   white / the color white

Examples:
   leukemia, leukocythemia (leuk/em/ia, leuk/o/cyt/hem/ia) — a frequently fatal condition in which there is an overproduction of white blood cells in the tissues (hem, em = blood)
   leukocyte (leuk/o/cyt/e) — a white (colorless) blood cell
   leukocyt- (leuk/o/cyt-) — combining form meaning white blood cell

Because there are so many morbid conditions characterized by an increase in the number of leukocytes in the blood, a variety of suffixes may be attached to this stem:
   leukocytosis (leuk/o/cyt/osis) — a condition of increased leukocytes in the blood
   leukocytoma (leuk/o/cyt/oma) — a tumorlike mass of leukocytes

lingua   tongue / the tongue; name for the tongue of the mouth

Examples:
   lingual (lingu/al) — pertaining to the tongue
   lingula (ling/ula) — a small tongue; generally a part of the body which is shaped like and projects like a tongue
   lingually (lingu/al/ly) — toward the tongue

This root means the same as gloss- (Lesson 3) in that both refer to the tongue in the mouth. However, they are used for different purposes. Lingu- is mostly used to designate the tongue as a structure, a point of reference (landmark):
   retrolingual (retr/o/lingu/al) — behind the tongue

Lesson 4 — Reading Assignment

Gloss- is the root which is principally used to denote diseases, injuries and the therapeutic procedures used for the alleviation of such diseases and injuries.

lobo-   section / a more or less well-defined portion of any organ, especially of the brain and glands

    Examples:
        lobe (lob/e) — name for a well-defined portion of an organ; organs having such parts are the brain, the lungs, the liver, the glands, the ears
        lobule (lob/ule) — a small lobe
        lobectomy (lob/ectomy) — excision of a lobe, as of the thyroid, liver, brain or lung
        lobar (lob/ar) — of or pertaining to a lobe or section

melan-   black / the color black

    Examples:
        melanin (melan/in) — a black or dark brown pigment in the skin and hair
        melanocyte (melan/o/cyt/e) — the cell responsible for the production of black pigment
        melanodermic, melanous (melan/o/derm/ic, melan/ous) — having a dark skin
        melanemia (melan/em/ia) — a condition in which the blood contains a black or dark brown pigment
        melanosis (melan/osis) — a condition characterized by abnormal deposits of black pigment; also called melan/ism
        cardiomelanosis (cardi/o/melan/osis) — deposits of black pigment in the heart; melanosis of the heart

myring-   eardrum / the sheet of membrane forming a partition between the outer and inner ear

    Examples:
        myringa (myring/a) — the eardrum; name of the eardrum
        myringoscopy (myring/o/scop/y) — inspection of the eardrum using a myringoscope
        myringoplasty (myring/o/plast/y) — surgical repair of defects of the eardrum

odont-   tooth

    Examples:
        odontic, odontal (odont/ic, odont/al) — pertaining to a tooth/pertaining to the teeth
        -odontia (-odont/ia) — form, condition or mode of treatment of the teeth
        odontogenic (odont/o/gen/ic) — originating in the teeth
        endodontics (end/odont/ics) — the branch of dentistry dealing with the inside of the tooth including the cause, prevention, diagnosis and treatment of diseases affecting the inner structure of a tooth, principally the pulp which fills the inside of the root canals; also called endodontia

semen   seed / the name of the thick, whitish secretion of the male reproductive organs which carries and transfers the sperm for fertilization of the egg in the female reproductive system

    Example:
        semenology (semen/ology) — the study of semen

    The root may also appear in the form **semin-**:
        seminal (semin/al) — pertaining to the semen
        semination (semin/ation) — introduction of semen into the genital tract of the female

spondyl-   spinal column or vertebra; vertebra, a bone of the spine; spinal column, the "back bone"

    This root is used to denote any one of the twenty-six bones (a vertebra; plural, the vertebrae) of the

Lesson 4 — Reading Assignment

back. It is also used to denote the spinal column which is the structure consisting of a series of jointed bones (vertebrae) beginning at the back of the head, extending through the neck and back and ending at the tailbone (which is the last of the vertebrae.)

Examples:
   spondylic, spondylous (spondyl/ic, spondyl/ous) — pertaining to a vertebra; pertaining to the spinal column

Spondyl-, in common with many of the other body parts which you have learned, can carry a variety of suffixes to denote morbid conditions or therapeutic procedures. Can you form the words which would mean "pain in," "inflammation of," "incision into," "any disease of," "puncture of"?

It's obvious that the column formed by these twenty-six bones must be jointed. Can you form the combination which would carry the meaning "inflammation of spinal joint(s)?"

steno-   narrow; contracted / constricted; close

This descriptive root can apply to a body structure to express less than normal width:
   stenocephalous (steno/cephal/ous) — having a narrow head
   stenocephalia (steno/cephal/ia) — excessive narrowness of the head
   stenostomia (steno/stom/ia) — narrowing of the mouth

Stenosis (steno/sis) is a word meaning constriction of a passage in the body such as a duct or canal thus producing a narrowing which interferes with passage of material through the tubelike passage.
   stenosis or -stenosis (steno/sis, -steno/sis) — narrowing of a duct or canal
   angiostenosis (angi/o/steno/sis) — narrowing of the diameter of a vessel
   enterostenosis (enter/o/steno/sis) — narrowing of the intestine

Stricture is a word which is also applied in medicine to denote abnormal narrowing of a canal, duct or passage either from the build up of healing tissue, such as a scar tissue, the deposit of normal tissue, inflammation (swelling) or as the result of a spasm.

trans-   through; across; beyond / to the other side

the "through" idea of the prefix trans- is encountered frequently in the description of operating techniques to describe the approach being made:
   transdermic (trans/derm/ic) — through the skin

The "across" idea is illustrated in actions involving a "movement across," a "carrying across," a "transfer":
   transfusion (trans/fus/ion) — (fus- means "to pour") the introduction of blood from another source; a "pouring across' of blood
   transplant (trans/plant) — a piece of tissue for grafting taken from another part of the patient's body or from a donor; a "planting across"

The "beyond" application, frequently carrying the idea of "more than," is seen in:
   transnormal (trans/normal) — beyond normal, more than normal

vaso-   vessel / any canal for carrying fluid; a duct; a channel; but, principally a blood vessel or lymph vessel

Here is another case in which we have two roots which are synonyms, vas- and angi- (Lesson 10, both of which mean vessel, especially a blood vessel. Although there is overlapping in their applications to medical terminology, for the most part, vas- is used in naming the various ailments affecting vessels and the therapy taken to overcome or correct such ailments.

Lesson 4 — Reading Assignment

Examples:

vascular (vas/cul/ar) — pertaining to a vessel; full of vessels

vasculum (vas/cul/um) — a small vessel

cerebrovascular (cerebr/o/vas/cul/ar) — pertaining to the blood vessels of the cerebrum or brain

myovascular (my/o/vas/cul/ar) — pertaining to the muscle and its blood vessels

vasectomy (vas/ectomy) — surgical excision of all or part of the duct in the male through which the sperm is secreted

Lesson 4 — Element Recognition Exercise

Separate the elements, connecting vowels, and word terminals of the following medical words by inserting a slash mark (/) between them.

Example: gastrolithiasis — gastr/o/lith/iasis

lobotomy

emetology

contraception

odontiasis

transdermic

bradyglossia

angiectasis

cytopathology

odontotripsis

leukocytopenia

hyperesthesia

cantholysis

stenocephaly

cheiloplasty

enterocele

semenologist

celialgia

erythrocyanosis

vasorrhaphy

melanocarcinoma

caudal

lingual

spondylodynia

leukoderma

canthorrhaphy

cheilitis

cystocele

celioma

erythropenia

vasalgia

melanoderma

myringoplasty

spondylolysis

lobectomy

lithiasis

transfusion

bradycardia

cardiectasis

cytogenesis

odontoptosis

cheilotomy

myringoscope

Lesson 5 — Review

ELEMENT	AUDIONYM	VISUAL IMAGE	MEANING
ovar- ova	over	See the **over**turned **egg** and **egg**s being turned **over**!	eggs (egg, the female reproductive cell)
-centesis	cent	See the **cent** being **puncture**d!	puncture
oto-	"O" toe	See the **"O" to**es with **ear**s!	ear
bili-	bill	See the **bill**s **pile**d high!	bile
squam-	squaw	See the **squa**w sitting on the **scale**!	scale
mening-	manage	See the **manage**r. She is **manag**ing **men**'s **brain**s!	membrane
cec-	seek	See the man **seek**ing the **passage** while **blind**folded!	blind passage
macul-	Mack (truck)	See the **Mack** truck with **spot**s all over it!	spot (or stain)
-pexy	pecks eggs	See the bird who **pecks** the **egg** while **suspended** and **fixed** in the air!	suspension, fixation
onco-	uncle	See the **uncle** being introduced; there are **two mor**e!	mass, tumor or swelling
or-	oar	See the **oar** with a **mouth** on it!	mouth
sub-	submarine	See the **sub**marine sandwich **under**, **beneath** or **below** the water!	under, beneath, below
spiro-	sparrow	See the **sparro**w with a **coil** head, **coil** tail, **coil** wings, **coil** feet!	coil

Lesson 5 — Review

ELEMENT	AUDIONYM	VISUAL IMAGE	MEANING
lacrim-	lake rim	See a **lake rim** crying a **tear!**	tear
viscero-	vice row	See the person on the **vice ro**wing with **organ**s!	organ
lact-	lacquer	See the **lac**quer being put on the furniture. Instead of lacquer, it is **milk**!	milk
onych-	onyx	See the **onyx** ring with a **nail** and a **claw** coming out of it!	nail, claw
thorac	throw rack	See the man **thro**wing a **rac**k attached to a treasure **chest**!	chest
pyle- pyloro-	pie	See the **pie** with a **gate** on it!	gate
vesic-	vest sick	See the **ves**t that is **sic**k. It is made of a **bladder**!	bladder
sphenic-	sphinx	See the **sphin**x made into a **wedge**!	wedge, wedge-shaped
myel-	mile	See the **mile** sign made of a **narrow spinal cord**!	marrow (Spinal cord)
anti-	ant eye	See the **ant** with its **eye against** the rock!	against
myco-	my comb	See **my co**mb with **fungus** all over it!	fungus
hallux-	hall "X"	See the **hall** shaped like an **"X"** with **great toe**s at the ends of the hall!	great toe (big toe)

Lesson 5 — Worksheet

Complete the following:

ELEMENT	AUDIONYM	MEANING
ovar-		
-centesis		
oto-		
bili-		
squam-		
mening-		
cec-		
macul-		
-pexy		
onco-		
or-		
sub-		
spiro-		
lacrim-		
viscero-		
lact-		
onych-		
thorac-		
pyle-pyloro-		
vesic-		
sphenic-		
myel-		
anti-		
myco-		
hallux-		

Lesson 5 — Word Terminals

-es   plural ending similar to **-s**

    Examples:
        kiss — kisses; fish — fishes; meninx (membrane) — meninges (membranes)

-id   pertaining to; "being"

    Examples:
        fluid (flu/id-) — to flow
        frigid (frig/id) — to be cold
        rigid (rig/id) — to be stiff
        parotid (par/ot/id) — being near the ear

-ness   state; quality; instance of being

    Examples:
        great/ness, sad/ness, together/ness, loneli/ness, good/ness, sick/ness

-us   noun ending; used to form the name of a thing from the root

    Example:
        disc/us

Lesson 5 — Reading Assignment

anti-   against / opposing; counteracting (acting against); inhibiting; preventing; suppressing; neutralizing or destroying; relieving

This prefix is widely used in medical terms as it is in common words with the broad meaning "against."

Examples:
    antigen (anti/gen) — a substance that, when introduced into the body, stimulates the "production of" an "opposing" substance called an anti/body
    antibody (anti/body) — a physical substance either in the body or produced by the action of an antigen which will prevent, relieve, or destroy the effect of infections or poisonous substances in the blood or tissues
    antacid (ant/acid) — a substance that counteracts or neutralizes acidity
    antiemetic (anti/emet/ic) — preventing or relieving nausea and vomiting
    anticoagulant (anti/coagulant) — a substance that suppresses or opposes the coagulation of the blood

bili-   bile / gall; a thick, sticky yellow or greenish fluid secreted by the liver and flowing into the intestines where it is mixed with gastric fluids to aid digestion, particularly in the breaking down of fats; chole-

Gallbladder, bile cyst, cholecyst — names for the sac or pouch in which bile is stored.

Examples:
    biliary (bili/ary) — pertaining to the bile or pertaining collectively to the bile, bile ducts and gallbladder

        biliary canal (bili/ary) — a tube (duct) through which the bile passes from the liver; hepatic duct; biliary duct
        biliary tract (bili/ary) — the region which secretes and transmits bile; the bile duct and gallbladder

    biliousness (bili/ous/ness) — a discomfort characterized by constipation, headache, and indigestion, attributed to an excess production of bile

cec-   a blind passage

A blind passage, like a "blind alley" is a space having only one outlet so that passage or flow cannot occur all the way through. Although the root may be used to refer to any such passage in the body, it is applied most frequently to denote the cecum.

The cecum (cec/um) is a large pouch at the beginning of the large intestine with only one opening. Incidentally, the appendix hangs at the end of the cecum.

As is true with other pouches in the body, the cecum may be:
    cut — cecotomy (cec/otomy)
    partially "cut out" — cecectomy (cec/ectomy)
    provided with a mouth or artificial opening — cecostomy (cec/ostomy)
    sutured — cecorrhaphy (cec/o/rrhaphy)
    fixed (usually to the abdominal wall) — cecopexy (cec/o/pexy)

The operations performed may be the result of conditions of disease or injury affecting the cecum:
    cecoptosis (cec/o/ptosis) — falling (downward displacement)
    cecitis (cec/itis) — inflammation

Lesson 5 — Reading Assignment

cecorrhexis (cec/o/rrhexis) — rupturing; the cecorrhexis may have produced a hernia (cec/o/cele)

cecal (cec/al) — pertaining to the cecum

-centesis   puncture / surgical puncture or incision, usually for the purpose of drainage

Examples:
arthrocentesis (arthr/o/centesis) — surgical puncture of a joint
cardicentesis (cardi/centesis) — surgical puncture or incision of the heart
pericardicentesis (peri/cardi/centesis) — surgical puncture of the tissues surrounding the heart (the pericardium)

hallux   great toe/big toe

This is the technical medical name for the big toe or the great toe; also called the first digit of the foot. The fingers and toes are called digits and are numbered from the great toe in the case of the foot and the thumb in the case of the hand. Thus, hallux = great toe = big toe = first digit of the foot which may be the first digit of the right foot (big toe of the right foot) or the first digit of the left foot (big toe of the left foot).

lacrim-   tear / the tears; tears of the eye

Examples:
lacrimal (sometimes lachrymal) (lacrim/al, lachrym/al) — pertaining to tears; relating to or situated near the organs that produce tears
lacrimal glands (lacrim/al) — the glands which secrete tears
lacrimal ducts (lacrim/al) — a term for ducts (canals, tubes) conveying the secretion (tears) of the lacrimal glands to the corner of the eye (canthus)
lacrimotomy (lacrim/otomy) — incision of the lacrimal duct

lact-   milk / the fluid secretion of the gland of the breast in the female forming the natural food of infants

Examples:
lacteal (lact/e/al) — pertaining to milk
lactation (lact/ation) — the secretion of milk; suckling by infants
lactogenic (lact/o/gen/ic) — stimulating the production of milk
lactigenous (lact/i/gen/ous) — producing or secreting milk
superlactation (super/lact/ation) — secretion of milk in greater than normal amount or for a longer than usual period

macul-   spot (or stain) / blotch; spotty or blotchy discoloration, especially of the skin

Examples:
macula (macul/a) — a spot or blotch
macule (macul/e) — a macula
maculation (macul/ation) — the condition of being spotted; the formation of spots or macules

Note: Tumors (-oma, onc-) are usually discolored but are always characterized by swelling. A macule is a discolored spot or patch which is flat, that is neither swollen or depressed. Birthmarks and freckles are examples of macules which are usually not a sign of disease. Macula, which are indicative of disease are the spots which appear in some of the infectious diseases such as smallpox and leprosy; psoriasis and some poisons also produce spotty discolorations.

mening-   membrane / the membranes covering the brain and the spinal cord (myel-)

Lesson 5 — Reading Assignment

Examples:

    meningeal (mening/e/al) — pertaining to the meninges

    meninges (mening/es) — name for the membranous sheath that envelops the brain and spinal cord

    meningoencephal- (mening/o/encephal-) — form for the meninges and the brain or the meninges and brainy substance

    meningitis (mening/itis) — inflammation of the membranes covering the brain and spinal cord (the meninges)

    cerebral meningitis (cerebr/al mening/itis) — inflammation of the meninges of the brain

myco-   fungus / relating to an infection with a fungus (a kind of plant which can form a destructive pathogen [disease producer] in humans and other animals)

Examples:

    mycete (myc/ete) — a fungus

    mycosis, -mycosis (myc/osis) — "a condition of fungus (infection)"; any disease caused by a fungus

    mycetoma, -mycetoma (myc/et/oma, -myc/et/oma) — a tumor containing fungus cells (mycetocytes)

    dermatomycosis (dermat/o/myc/osis) — a fungus infection of the skin which includes the conditions commonly called "athlete's foot" and "ring worm"

    acromycosis (acr/o/myc/osis) — a condition of fungus infection of the extremities (limbs)

myel-   marrow (spinal cord) / the soft inner part of a bone; the cablelike tissue enclosed in the canal or tube formed by the bones of the spine (the vertebrae)

Examples:

    meningomyel- (mening/o/myel-) form for the spinal cord and its membranous covering; also myel/o/mening/o-

    osteomyel- (oste/o/myel-) — form for bone marrow or the bone and its marrow

    osteomyelitis (oste/o/myel/itis) — inflammation of the bone and the bone marrow

    encephalomyel- (en/cephal/o/myel-) — form for the brain and the spinal cord; also myel/o/en/cephal-

    encephalomyelopathy (en/cephal/o/myel/o/path/y) — any disease or diseased condition of the brain and spinal cord

    myeloencephalitis (myel/o/en/cephal/itis) — inflammation of the brain and spinal cord

Note: The marrow of the bone and the spinal cord have structural similarities in that they are both surrounded by bone: bone marrow being the soft tissue filling the hollow interior of a bone; the spinal cord being a covered (mening-) "cable" of nerve fibers and tissues which runs through the hollowed centers of the stack of vertebrae forming the spine.

onco-   mass, tumor, swelling

Examples:

    -oncus (-onc/us) — designation for a swelling or tumor

    arthroncus (arthr/onc/us) — swelling of a joint

    blepharoncus (blephar/onc/us) — tumor on the eyelid

    cheiloncus (cheil/onc/us) — a tumor of the lip

    glossoncus (gloss/onc/us) — a swelling of the tongue

    mastoncus (mast/onc/us) — a tumor of the breast or mammary gland

onych-   nail; claw / a fingernail, a toenail

Lesson 5 — Reading Assignment

Examples:
-onychium (-onych/ium) — region of the fingernail or toenail
eponychium (ep/onych/ium) — the cuticle; the narrow band of skin (epidermis) that extends from the nail wall onto the nail surface
-onychia (-onych/ia) — a condition of the nails of the fingers or toes
leukonychia (leuk/onych/ia) — whitish spots or discoloration of the nails
   Sometimes -onychia is used to indicate inflammation in or around the nails.
onychia (onych/ia) — inflammation of the nail bed (matrix) resulting in the loss of the nail
eponychia (ep/onych/ia) — inflammation of the cuticle of the nail

or-   mouth / the mouth; the body structure bounded at the front by the lips and containing the tongue and teeth

This root is seen in the well-known word **oral** meaning "pertaining to the mouth."

Examples:
orad (or/ad) — toward the mouth
circumoral (circum/or/al) — the area around the mouth (**circum** means around as in circumference, the distance around a circle)

Note: Or- is used to designate the mouth as an anatomical part; stom-, stomat- is used to designate disease, injuries and therapy on the mouth.

oto-   ear / the ear

Because the ear is such a prominent feature of the head, it is used, not only for conditions which affect the ear, e.g. pain (ot/algia), water in the ear (hydr/ot/is), inflammation (ot/itis), but also as a landmark for use in locating other body parts which are less visible; this is indicated by the suffix stem -otic (-ot/ic) or -otid (-ot/id).

Examples:
parotid (par/ot/id) — situated near the ear such as the parotid gland, a salivary gland located near the ear
epiotic (epi/ot/ic) — situated on or above the ear
entotic or endotic (ent/ot/ic or end/ot/ic) — situated in or arising in the ear

ovar-   egg (the female reproductive gland) / the paired female reproductive organ that produces eggs and female sex hormones

The root ov- means "egg" and forms the medical words:
ovum (ov/um) — to denote the female reproductive cell which, upon fertilization after encountering semen- (see Lesson 4), begins the process of reproduction (the production of offspring)
ova (ov/a) — "eggs," the plural of ovum

The combination of elements in ov/ar- literally means "place for the ova" or, more familiarly, "an egg container."

Examples:
ovary (ov/ar/y) — name for the sexual gland in the female in which the ova are formed
ovariogenic (ovari/o/gen/ic) — produced in or arising in the ovary
ovariocentesis (ovari/o/centesis) — surgical puncture of an ovary

-pexy   suspension; fixation / the surgical act of fastening or making firm or solid

When organs are displaced (-ptosis), the surgical operation to repair this condition by restoring the

Lesson 5 — Reading Assignment

organ to its proper place is called "fixation" or "suspension." The suffix -pexy is used to denote this procedure and may be interpreted as "surgical fixation of."

Examples:
    nephropexy (nephr/o/pexy) — surgical fixation of the kidney
    gastropexy (gastr/o/pexy) — surgical fixation of the stomach
    hysteropexy (hyster/o/pexy) — surgical fixation of the womb

pyle-, pyloro-   gate / a "gate," an opening, a passage

These elements have a basic root pyl- which carries the meaning "gate" or "opening."

The root pyle- is used for relationships to an important vein, the portal vein, which is a large vein carrying blood from the digestive organs and the spleen to the liver.
    pylic (pyl/ic) — pertaining to the portal vein

the root pylor- which literally means "gate keeper" is used for relationships to the pylorus which is the opening of the stomach into the intestines through which the stomach contents pass into the intestines.
    pyloric (pylor/ic) — pertaining to the pylorus
    gastropylor- (gastr/o/pylor) — form for the stomach and the pylorus

        gastropyloric (gastr/o/pylor/ic) — pertaining to the stomach and the pylorus
        gastropylorectomy (gastr/o/pylor/ectomy) — excision of the pyloric portion of the stomach

sphenic   a wedge; wedge-shaped

Examples:
    sphenoid (sphen/oid) — resembling a wedge; in the shape of a wedge
    sphenoid bone (sphen/oid) — an irregular wedge-shaped bone at the base of the cranium
    sphenocephaly (sphen/o/cephal/y) — a developmental abnormality characterized by a wedge-shaped appearance of the head

spiro-   coil / a coil- a winding, twisting

Examples:
    spiroid (spir/oid) — resembling a spiral or coil
    spiradeno- (spir/aden/o-) — a form used interchangeably with hidradeno- (hidr/aden/o) to denote a sweat gland; so called because of the spiral shape of a sweat gland

Spiro- should not be confused with **spir-** appearing in words as perspire (per/spir/e), perspiration (per/spir/ation), aspiration (a/spir/ation), respiration (re/spir/ation). In these the element means "breath" or "breathing."

squam-   scale / a scale, a platelike structure (such as scales and scaly structure on a fish)

Examples:
    squama (squam/a) — a scale or platelike structure
    squamous, squamosa (squam/ous, squam/osa) — scaly or platelike
    squamate (squam/ate) — scaly; having or resembling scales

The rough skin which peels as a result of sunburn is an example of squama.
Squamous carcinoma (also squamous cell carcinoma) is skin cancer.

sub-   under, beneath, below / less than

Lesson 5 — Reading Assignment

Examples:
    subdermal (sub/derm/al) — situated or occurring under the skin
    subnormal (sub/norm/al) — below or less than normal
    sublingual (sub/lingu/al) — located beneath the tongue; also subglossal
    subinflammation (sub/inflammation) — a slight or mild inflammation (sub = below, less than, slight or mild)
    submania (sub/man/ia) — mania of a moderate type; also hypomania

thorac-   chest / the part of the body situated between the neck and the abdomen and supported by the cagelike structure formed by the ribs

Examples:
    thorax — medical name for the chest; also called thorac/ic cavity
    thoracic (thorac/ic) — (sometimes thor/ac/al) — pertaining to the chest
    thoracogastr- (thorac/o/gastr-) — relating to the stomach and chest (thorax)
    thoracicoabdominal (thorac/ic/o/abdomin/al) — pertaining to the chest and the abdomen
    suprathoracic (supra/thorac/ic) — situated above the thorax
    hemothorax (hem/o/thorax) — a collection of blood in the lung cavity

vesic-   bladder / a bladder; the urinary bladder

Examples:
    vesica (vesic/a) — general term for a bladder
    vesical (vesic/al) — pertaining to (principally) the urinary bladder
    vesico- (vesic/o) — form relating to a bladder or the urinary bladder
    vesicle — medical name for a small bladder, sac or blister containing liquid
    vesicula (vesic/ul/a) — general term used in anatommical nomenclature for a vesicle (small sac or bladder)
    vesicular (vesic/ul/ar) — (1) formed or constructed like a small sac or bladder; (2) containing, made up of, or characterized by small saclike bodies

Vesic- compared with cyst-: Again we have two roots which have the same meaning but are applied differently. Vesic- is the root generally used in naming the various bladders or bladder-like structures in the body; cyst- is the root generally used in naming of diseases and therapeutic procedures involving bladders or bladder- like structures.

viscero-   organ / an internal organ or the internal organs of the body especially those located in the large cavity of the trunk such as the heart, the liver, the intestines, etc.

Examples:
    visceral (viscer/al) — pertaining to an internal organ, especially those in the abdomen
    viscera (viscer/a) — name for internal organs taken collectively, especially those in the abdomen
    viscerad (viscer/ad) — toward the viscera
    visceroptosis (viscer/o/ptosis) — a dropping or falling down of the viscera due, for example, to the weakness of the abdominal muscles

Lesson 5 — Element Recognition Exercise

Separate the elements, connecting vowels, and word terminals of the following medical words by inserting a slash mark (/) between them.

Example: pylorogastrectomy — pyloro/gastr/ectomy

ovigenesis

thoracentesis

otolithiasis

bilious

squamous

meningocerebritis

cecopexy

macula

nephropexy

oncosis

oralogy

subcutaneous

myelomalacia

spiroid

lacrimotomy

visceroptosis

lactigenous

onychomalacia

thoracomyodynia

pylorostenosis

vesicocele

myelomeningitis

antimycotic

mycomyringitis

oncology

subglossitis

visceralgia

lactocele

onychorrhexis

thoracoscopy

mycosis

antiplastic

hepatopexy

cecum

sphenoidotomy

vesicotomy

ovoid

arthrocentesis

otodynia

biligenesis

meningeorrhaphy

sphenocephaly

Lesson 6—Review

ELEMENT	AUDIONYM	VISUAL IMAGE	MEANING
physio-	physics book	See the **physi**cs book with a **nature** boy streaking out of it!	nature
bucc(o)-	bucket	See the **buc**ket with **cheeks** on it!	cheek
palpebr-	pile of people	See the **pile** of **pe**ople with very large **eyelids**!	eyelid
plasia-	play show	See the **pla**y **sh**ow **developing** film!	development or growth
rug-	rug	See the **rug** with **wrinkle**s, **fold**s, and **crease**s in it!	wrinkle, fold, crease
aur-	"R"	See the **"R"** with an **ear** on it!	ear
acoust(i)-	a cue stick	See **a cue sti**ck with a **hearing** aid on it and **sound** coming out of it!	hearing, sound
colp(o)-	cold bow	See the **col**d **bo**w that is **hollow** with a **Virginia** ham inside of it!	hollow, vagina
phon-	phone	See the **phon**e with **voice** and **sound** coming out of it although no one is using it!	voice, sound
leio-	lei	See the **lei** with all the flowers gone. It is **smooth**!	smooth
cor	core	See the apple **cor**e with the **heart** inside of it!	heart
ren-	rain	See it **rain**ing **kid**s on their **knee**s!	kidney

Lesson 6 — Review

ELEMENT	AUDIONYM	VISUAL IMAGE	MEANING
orchi-	orchid	See the **orchi**d with **tests** in it!	testis
encephal-	hen sieve fall	See the h**en** in a **sieve fall**ing. It has a **brain** instead of a head!	brain
thalam-	the lamb	See **the lam**b who was the w**inner** of the **Chamber** of Commerce Contest!	inner chamber
plexus	plexiglass	See **plexi**glass with **braid**s hanging down in front of it!	braid, an interweaving or network
cilia	ceiling	See the **ceili**ng with **eyelash**es!	eyelash
dendr-	den door	See the **den d**oor in the **tree** with **branches**!	tree, branching (as in nervous system)
phleb-	flip flipchart	See the **flip**chart with **vein**s all over it!	vein
pilo-	pile on	See the man **pil**ing **on hair** on another man's head. He piles it on and piles it on!	hair
histo-	his toe	See **his to**e with **tissue**s coming out of it!	tissue
stoma-	stone	See the **sto**ne with a **mouth** on it!	mouth or opening
tympan-	tin pan	See inside the **tin pan**. It has an **ear** on a **drum**!	eardrum or its enclosure
umbilic-	a bill lick	See **a bill** being **lic**ked with a **naval** officer coming out of it!	navel
salpingo-	Sally Bingo	See **Sal**ly playing **Bingo** while sitting in an inner **tube**!	tube

Lesson 6 — Worksheet

Complete the following:

ELEMENT	AUDIONYM	MEANING
physio-		
bucc(o)-		
palpebr-		
plasia-		
rug-		
aur-		
acoust(i)-		
colp(o)-		
phon-		
leio-		
cor		
ren-		
orchi-		
encephal-		
thalam-		
plexus		
cilia		
dendr-		
phleb-		
pilo-		
histo-		
stoma-		
tympan-		
umbilic-		
salpingo-		

Lesson 6 — Word Terminals

-ian   (one) belonging to or having some relation to; one believing in or following

Examples:
Christ/ian, Grec/ian, Ind/ian, Florid/ian, Pennsylvan/ian
(same as *-an*, see Lesson 2)

-ism   an abnormal condition

This terminal is similar in meaning to *-osis.*

Examples:
alcohol/ism, morphin/ism, mongol/ism

-ite   a part of the body or bodily organ

Example:
dendrite (dendr/ite) — a body part characterized by its appearance of branching

-itic   pertaining to or affected by inflammation

This terminal is a combination of *-itis* (Lesson 1) and *-ic* ("pertaining to", Reading Assignment, Lesson 1) and is used to refer to a condition of inflammation.

Examples:
arthr/itic, gastr/itic, nephr/itic

-on   noun ending; used to form the name of a thing from the root

Example:

en/cephal/on

Lesson 6 — Reading Assignment

acoust(i)-   hearing; sound

Examples:
    acoustic (acoust/ic) — pertaining to hearing
    acoustogram (acoust/o/gram) — the graphic tracing of the measures of sound such as decibel levels and frequency per second

Because of the familiarity of acousti- in words for sound, we have chosen to present the root in this form. However, the basic root meaning sound is ***acous-*** or ***acus-***.

    -acusis (-acu/sis) — used to denote a condition of hearing (also -acusia)
    anacusis (an/acu/sis) — "condition of not hearing"; total deafness (an- means "not" and is discussed in Lesson 10)
    hemianacusia (hemi/an/acus/ia) — loss of hearing in one ear only

aur-   ear

Examples:
    auricle (aur/i/cle) — the projecting part of the ear lying outside the head
    auricul-) aur/i/cul) — form denoting relationship to the ear or to an ear-shaped appendage of a chamber of the heart
    auriculocranial (aur/i/cul/o/crani/al) — pertaining to an ear and the cranium
    auris (aur/is) — the ear

The element ***oto-***, ear, (Lesson 5) is the more widely used form for denoting conditions of the ear and the therapeutic procedures to correct such conditions.

bucc(o)-   cheek

Examples:
    buccal (bucc/al) — pertaining to the cheek; directed toward the cheek
    buccally (bucc/al/ly) — toward the cheek

This root is used widely as a landmark or point of reference in locating other (usually less prominent) structures or features of other structures. For example, in dentistry the buccal surface of a tooth is the surface on the side toward the cheek.
    buccocervical (bucc/o/cervic/al) — that surface of a tooth along its neckline (the part of the tooth at the point where it enters the gum) on the cheek side
    suprabuccal (supra/bucc/al) — above the cheek region

cilia   eyelash / the lashes of the eye; also a hairlike projection

Examples:
    ciliary (cili/ary) — pertaining to the eyelashes; resembling the eyelashes
    cilium (cili/um) — the eyelashes; also sometimes the eyelid or the outer edge of the eyelid or the edge of the eyelid from which the eyelashes extend
    supercilia (super/cilia) — the eyebrows (super- is a prefix that is close in meaning to supra- [Lesson 3]; here it means "above"). Literally, then, the meaning is "above the eyelashes."
    ciliogenesis (cili/o/gen/esis) — the formation or development of cilia

colp(o)-   hollow; vagina / the canal in the female which forms a passage from the uterus to the outside of the body

Examples:
    -colpos (-colp/os) — suffix stem used to denote a vaginal disorder of a specific type, such as:

Lesson 6 — Reading Assignment

pyocolpos (py/o/colp/os) — collection of pus within the vagina
hematocolpos (hemat/o/colp/os) — an accumulation of menstrual blood in the vagina

colpitis (colp/itis) — inflammation of the vagina

Note: Vagin- is also a root used to denote relationships to any sheathlike structure, but especially the vagina as defined above.
vaginal (vagin/al) — pertaining to the vagina; of the nature of a sheath

cor   heart / the heart / the muscular organ that maintains the circulation of the blood

This is a word used in international nomenclature to denote the heart. It is introduced to mark a distinction from the element **coron-** meaning "crown" which is often used broadly to indicate the heart and **cardi-** which is the most widely used root to name conditions of the heart and therapeutic procedures applied to the heart.

Another form in which **cor** appears is **cord-** in such words as:

cordate (cord/ate) — heart-shaped
cordial (cord/i/al) — stimulating the heart

dendr-   tree; branching (as in the nervous system)

This descriptive root which can be interpreted as "branching" is used to describe body structures or parts resembling the branching of a tree; especially used for the nerve fibers that extend from a nerve cell (dendrite).

Examples:
dendrite (dendr/ite) — name for the nerve fibers that extend from a nerve cell
dendritic (dendr/it/ic) — resembling a dendrite; branching like a tree
dendroid (dendr/oid) — branching like a tree

encephal-   brain

Examples:
encephalic (en/cephal/ic) — pertaining to the brain; also, lying within the cranial cavity
encephalon (en/cephal/on) — name for the brain

The element **cephal** was introduced in Lesson 3; however, because of the frequent use of **en-cephal-** in medical terminology, we have introduced **encephal-** as an element in order that you might more easily remember the "brain" meaning of encephal-.

histo-   tissue / a mass of cells that forms one of the structural materials out of which the body is built up; a weblike structure

An important clue for recognizing words dealing with tissues is the word ending **-ium** (sometimes -eum). Many (probably most) of the words you encounter having an -ium (or -eum) ending denote tissues:
endocardium (end/o/card/ium) — the tissue (membrane) lining the heart
endosteum (end/ost/eum) — the tissue lining the cavity of a bone and surrounding the bone marrow

Examples:
histocyte (hist/o/cyt/e) — a tissue cell
histoma (hist/oma) — a tumor formed from fully developed tissue such as blood vessels, muscles, etc.

Lesson 6 — Reading Assignment

histolysis (hist/o/lysis) — the breaking down and destruction of tissue

histology (hist/ology) — the study (usually microscopic) of the structure, composition and functions of the tissues

leio-   smooth / especially, the "smooth" or "involuntary" muscles

This descriptive root may be used in reference to any smooth surface; it is especially used in the description of tumors to distinguish the so called "smooth" muscles which are generally found in the walls of the stomach, intestines, vessels and glands; they are also in the very small muscles of the skin and, when contracted, produce what is called "goose flesh." The "smooth muscles" are also called "involuntary muscles" because they are not under control of the will.

Examples:
   leiomyoma (lei/my/oma) — a tumor composed of smooth muscle fibers
   leiodermia (leio/derm/ia) — abnormal glossiness or smoothness of the skin

orchi-   testis / testicle; one of the two male reproductive glands

Examples:
   orchic, orchidic (orch/ic, orchid/ic) — pertaining to the testicles
   -orchidism, -orchism (-orchid/ism, -orch/ism) — a (specified) form or condition of the testes
   orchitis (orch/itis) — inflammation of a testicle
   orchidopexy (orchid/o/pexy) — the surgical fixing in place of a displaced testicle

palpebr-   eyelid

Examples:
   palpebral (palpebr/al) — pertaining to an eyelid
   palpebra (palpebr/a) — the eyelid
   palpebrate (palpebr/ate) — to wink
   palpebration (palpebr/ation) — abnormally frequent winking

Here is another root meaning "eyelid." The tendency to use **palpebr-** as the root for naming or referring to the eyelid as an anatomical part; **blephar-** is the root used principally for the naming of conditions and therapeutic procedures involving the eyelid.

phleb-   vein / one of the branching blood vessels that carries blood toward the heart (compared to arteries which carry blood away from the heart)

Examples:
   phlebectasis (phleb/ectasis) — an enlargement (dilatation) of a vein; also phlebectasia
   phlebolith (phleb/o/lith) — "vein stone"; a bloodclot, in a vein, which has turned chalky
   phlebostenosis (phleb/o/sten/osis) — narrowing or constriction of a vein
   phlebophlebostomy (phleb/o/phleb/ostomy) — surgical openings to provide communication between two veins
   phlebitis (phleb/itis) — inflammation of a vein

phon-   voice; sound

This description root is generally used to denote speech or body sounds; the body sounds may be those arising within the body (heart beats) or created by such means as percussion (tapping)

Examples:
   phonic, phonal (phon/ic, phon/al) — pertaining to the voice

Lesson 6 — Reading Assignment

phonocardiogram (phon/o/cardi/o/gram) — a record of heart sounds
phonogram (phon/o/gram) — a record of any sound
phonomyogram (phon/o/my/o/gram) — a record of the sound produced by muscle action
phonopathy (phon/o/path/y) — any disease or disorder of the organs of speech

physio-   nature / the body (frequently as opposed to the mind)

Examples:
physiology (physi/ology) — the study of the functions of the body and its parts

pathologic physiology (path/o/log/ic physi/ology) — the study of disordered function or of function in diseased tissue
general physiology (physi/ology) — the study of the general laws of life and functional activity

physiatrics (phys/iatr/ics) — the diagnosis and treatment of disease with the aid of physical agents such as light, heat, cold, water, and electricity, or with mechanical apparatus
physician (phys/ic/ian) — an authorized practitioner of medicine

attending physician (phys/ic/ian) — a physician who attends a hospital at stated times to visit the patients and give direction as to their treatment
resident physician (phys/ic/ian) — a graduate and licensed physician resident in a hospital

pilo-   hair

Examples:
pilus (pil/us) — a hair
pilous, pilose, pileous, pilosity (pil/ous, pil/ose, pil/eous, pil/os/ity) — hairiness, covered with hair
pilosis (pil/osis) — excessive growth of hair
pilocystic (pil/o/cyst/ic) — cystlike and containing hair; used to describe certain skin tumors
depilation (depil/ation) — the process of removing hair; the agent for hair removal is a depilatory (the prefix de- has a meaning "remove" as in the familiar words de/hydr/ate, de/magnetize, de/contaminate, etc.)

-plasia   development or growth

Examples:
hyperplasia (hyper/plasia) — abnormal increase in growth; usually applied to abnormal increase in the cells making up tissues
hypoplasia (hypo/plasia) — incomplete or defective development
mastoplasia (mast/o/plasia) — the development of breast tissue

plexus   braid, an interweaving or network / a network or tangle used in medical (anatomical) terminology to designate a network of lymphatic vessels, nerves or veins

Examples:
plexal (plex/al) — pertaining to a plexus
plexiform (plex/i/form) — resembling a plexus or network
subplexal (sub/plex/al) — situated beneath a plexus or network of vessels, nerves or veins

ren-   kidneys / a kidney; the glandular bodies in the lower back which secrete urine (also nephr-)

Example:
renal (ren/al) — pertaining to the kidney

ren- vs. nephr-: The root **ren-** is used principally as a landmark, that is, a point of reference in locating other nearby structures:

Lesson 6 — Reading Assignment

supraren- (supra/ren-) — situated above the kidney, especially with reference to the suprarenal gland

The root **nephr-** is used principally to name the conditions affecting the kidneys (diseases, symptoms, etc.) and the surgical procedures performed on the kidney.

rug-   wrinkle; fold; crease

Examples:
   ruga (rug/a) — a ridge, wrinkle or fold, as of mucous membrane
   rugose, rugous (rug/ose, rug/ous) — characterized by wrinkles
   rugosity (rug/osity) — the condition of being wrinkled; a fold, ridge or wrinkle

salpingo-   tube / any tube or trumpet-shaped structure, especially the uterine tube into which the ovum (egg cell) passes when it leaves the ovary (egg case); also the auditory (hearing) tube

The element salping- might better be remembered as tuba-like since, like a tuba, it is a tube which is flared at the end. The name for such a tube (or tuba-like) structure is salpinx. there are two important structures in the body having this shape:

   The fallopian tubes (also called uterine tubes): two tubes in the reproductive system of the female which transmit the ovum (eggs) to the uterus (womb) and in which fertilization (conception) begins.

   The eustachian tube: tube in the ear which extends from the ear to the throat and is the means of equalizing pressure within the inner ear with the pressure of the atmosphere. When pressure builds on the tympanic membrane (changes in altitude such as airplane and elevator ascents and descents), relief is obtained by equalizing this pressure by yawning, swallowing, or nose-blowing which relieves the pressure difference in the eustachian tube. Also called the hearing tube and auditory tube.

Examples:
   salpingostomy (salping/ostomy) — the making (by surgery) of an opening into the fallopian (uterine) tube because the natural opening has become closed
   endosalpinx (end/o/salpin/x) — the mucous membrane lining the salpinx (the fallopian or uterine tube)

stoma-   mouth or opening / the mouth of the face

In Lesson 2 you learned the root **stoma-** in the form **-ostomy**, a mouthlike opening which is derived from stoma.

The root may appear in the form stomat-:
   stomatology (stomat/ology) — the branch of medicine which treats of the mouth and its disease
   stomatoplasty (stomat/o/plast/y) — plastic surgery of, operative repair of, defects of the mouth
   stomatogastric (stomat/o/gastr/ic) — pertaining to the stomach and the mouth
   stomatalgia (stomat/algia) — "mouth pain"; pain in the mouth; also stom/algia

thalam-   inner chamber / large gray mass which is part of the brain

Examples:
   thalamus (thalam/us) — name for the large gray mass in the brain
   thalamic (thalam/ic) — pertaining to the thalamus

This root is used in medical terminology to show relations to the thalamus, the part of the brain

Lesson 6 — Reading Assignment

which serves as a "switchboard" for the relaying of "messages." It is in this section that sensations such as pain, smell, touch are correlated with the taking of actions.

The root is used principally as a landmark. The thalam/us, epi/thalam/us, hypo/thalam/us, and sub/thalam/us are terms applied to name the parts (chambers) of a large brain cavity called the di/en/cephal/on (di- is a prefix meaning "two").

tympan-   eardrum or its enclosure

Examples:
    tympanum (tympan/um) — name for the enclosure or chamber in which the eardrum is located; also called the tympanic cavity
    tympanic membrane (tympan/ic) — name for the eardrum
    tympanal (tympan/al) — pertaining to the tympanum (the tympanic cavity); pertaining to the tympanic cavity (the eardrum)
    tympanic (tympan/ic) — pertaining to the tympanum (the tympanic cavity)

umbilic-   navel / "belly button"

Examples:
    umbilicus (umbilic/us) — name for the navel ("belly button")
    umbilical (umbilic/al) — pertaining to the umbilicus or navel
    umbilicectomy (umbilic/ectomy) — excision of the umbilicus
    parumbilical (par/umbilic/al) — near the navel

Lesson 6 — Element Recognition Exercise

Separate the elements, connecting vowels, and word terminals of the following medical words by inserting a slash mark (/) between them.

Example: encephalomyelitis — en/cephal/o/myel/itis

physiolysis

buccogingival

palpebritis

colpohyperplasia

auriscope

acoustic

colpoceliocentesis

phonocardiogram

leiomyoma

renotrophic

orchidoptosis

encephalomalacia

ciliogenesis

dendroid

phlebolithiasis

pilosis

histoid

stomatoplasty

tympanectomy

salpingostomy

leiodermia

renicardiac

orchiomyeloma

encephalolith

ciliectomy

phleborrhexis

pilology

histolysis

stomatomalacia

tympanotomy

umbilectomy

salpingocele

physiology

buccolingual

palpebral

hypoplasia

colpectasis

phonopathy

stomatalgia

salpingitis

histoma

colporrhaphy

Lesson 7 — Review

ELEMENT	AUDIONYM	VISUAL IMAGE	MEANING
helio-	heel	See the **heel** with the **sun** bursting out of it!	sun, light
astr-	astronaut	See the **astr**onaut with the **star shaped** head!	star shaped
-asthenia	his thin knee	See **his thin knee** with a **week**ly calendar tied around it!	weakness
fascia	face	See the **face** with a **sheet** over it and the **band** marching out over it!	sheet, band
iso-	I sew	See the lady saying, "**I sew** with **a quail**" as she sews with the quail!	equal
tarso-	tar	See the **tar** with a **triangle** stuck into it!	ankle region — instep
-tope	top	See the **top** spinning with a **place**mat on top of it!	place
pod-	pod	See the **pod** with a **foot** in it instead of peas!	foot
malign-	my leg	See **my leg** made out of a baseball **bat**!	bad, harmful
adnexa-	annex	See the **annex** being **tie**d to the main building!	ties, connections
ocul-	a "Kool"	See the image of "**a Kool**" with an **eye** on it!	eye
lapar-	lap	See the **lap** with an **apple** on the **wall**!	abdominal wall
dacry-	daiquiri	See the **daiquiri** cocktail crying a **tear**!	tear

Lesson 7 — Review

ELEMENT	AUDIONYM	VISUAL IMAGE	MEANING
ment-	mint	See the people pulling the **mint** saying, **"Mine! Mine!"**!	mind
part-	part	See the **part** in the hair with the **labor**er **bring**ing **forth** a two by four!	labor, bring forth
scler(a)-	scholar	See the **sch**olar wearing the **hard** hat!	hard
somato-	sew my toe	See the man saying, 'I'll **sew my toe** onto my **body**"!	body
trachel-	tray coal	See the **tray** with **coal** and a **neck** coming up through it!	neck or necklike structure
sinus	sign us	See the two men saying, "**sign us** in the **hollow space**"!	hollow space
hypno-	hypnotist	See the **hypno**tist who put himself to **sleep**!	sleep
sept-	sipped	See the person **sip**ping a drink through the **wall** with a **fence** on it!	wall, fence
scirr(h)-	skirt	See the **skir**t with **hard** hats all over it!	hard
antr-	ant tree	See the **ant** in a tree falling into a **cave-in** (cavity)!	cavity or chamber
-crine	cry'n	See the person **cry'n** to **see** the **crate**!	to secrete
dura	door	See the **door** with **hard** hats all over it!	hard

Lesson 7 — Worksheet

Complete the following:

ELEMENT	AUDIONYM	MEANING
helio-		
astr-		
-asthenia		
fascia		
iso-		
tarso-		
-tope		
pod-		
malign-		
adnexa-		
ocul-		
lapar-		
dacry-		
ment-		
part-		
scler(a)-		
somato-		
trachel-		
sinus		
hypno-		
sept-		
scirr(h)-		
antr-		
-crine		
dura		

Lesson 7 — Word Terminals

-ance, -ancy   a state or condition; the act of

Examples:
brilliance (brilli/ance) — the state or condition of being brilliant
elegance (eleg/ance) — the state or condition of being elegant
assistance (assist/ance) — the act of assisting
resistance (resist/ance) — the act of resisting

-ition   (same meaning as **-ation**, see Word Terminals, Lesson 4) a process, action or condition

Examples:
addition (add/ition) — the process of adding
prohibition (prohib/ition) — the act of denying, prohibiting
ambition (amb/ition) — a state of striving for achievement

-ician   of or belonging to; frequently, a person belonging to or associated with

This terminal is a combination of **-ic** (Word Terminals, Lesson 1) and **-ian** (see **-an**, **-ian**, Word Terminals, Lesson 2) and carries the same meaning as **-an**, **-ian**

Examples:
techni/cian, electr/ician, phys/ician, mathemat/ician

Lesson 7 — Reading Assignment

adnexa   ties; connections / appendages or adjacent parts

This word is a combination of a prefix **ad-** meaning "to" plus the root **nex-** meaning "join." Literally, the word means "joined to" and is applied chiefly to refer to the ocular adnexa, the appendages to the eye such as the lacrimal apparatus and the uterine adnexa, the appendages or adjacent parts to the womb such as the ovaries, the uterine tubes and the ligaments.

Examples:
   adnexopexy (adnex/o/pexy) — the operation of fixing the uterine adnexa to the abdominal walls
   adnexitis (adnex/itis) — inflammation of the uterine adnexa

antr-   cavity or chamber / a sinus; a hollow space; a cavity

Examples:
   antrum (antr/um) — a sinus; a cavity or chamber, especially within a bone
   antral (antr/al) — pertaining to a sinus or an antrum

The words antrum and sinus are synonyms in most applications. Generally, **sinus** is used to name a cavity or chamber as, for example, nasal sinus or nasal sinuses. **Antr-** is more frequently used as a root in forming single words relating to sinuses or antrums.

Examples:
   antrostomy (antr/ostomy) — the operation of making an opening into an antrum for the purpose of drainage
   antrodynia (antr/odyn/ia) — pain in an antrum

-asthenia   weakness / lack of strength, "not strong"

This suffix combination is formed from three useful elements, the prefix **a-** meaning "not" or "lacking" plus the root **sthen-** meaning "strength" or "strong" plus the word ending **-ia** meaning "morbid (diseased) condition." Literally, the combination can be translated as "a condition of lacking strength" or "weakness."

Preceeding elements are added to provide more information, such as:
   adenasthenia (aden/asthenia) — a weakness in glandular secretion; deficient glandular activity
   gastric adenasthenia (gastr/ic aden/asthenia) — deficient glandular secretion in the stomach

Asthen- may also be used with the same meaning "lacking strength" or "weakness."
   asthenia (asthen/ia) — lack or loss of strength and energy; weakness
   asthenic (asthen/ic) — pertaining to or characterized by asthenia
   asthenopia (asthen/op/ia) — a condition of weakness in the eye

astr-   star-shaped / resembling a star in form

Examples:
   astrocyte (astr/o/cyt/e) — a star-shaped cell, especially such a cell of the supporting structure of nervous tissue
   astroid (astr/oid) — star-shaped
   astrocytoma (astr/o/cyt/oma) — a tumor composed of star-shaped cells (astrocytes)

-crine   to secrete

This word ending which is used to indicate secretions of body fluids is most prominent in medical terminology in naming the endocrine system, the "secreting into" system. The endocrine system is made up of the endocrine glands which secrete the substance hormone into the blood stream. The endocrine system, in conjunction with the nervous system, carries on the activities of the body. Some of the endocrine glands and the functions they perform are:

thyroid gland — growth and metabolism
pituitary gland — skeletal growth
adrenal gland — responds to need for increased body activity under stress
gonads — the female ovaries and the male testes

Examples:

crinogenic (crin/o/gen/ic) — stimulating (producing) secretion
hypocrinia, also called hypocrinism (hypo/crin/ia, hypo/crin/ism) — deficient secretion of any endocrine gland
hypercrinia, also called hypercrinism (hyper/crin/ia, hyper/crin/ism) — excessive secretion of any endocrine gland

dacry-   tear / tear of the eye

In Lesson 5 we learned that **lacrim-** is a root also meaning tear or tears of the eye. The root **lacrim-** is generally used to denote the body parts or structures having to do with the production of tears. Conditions relating to tear production are generally denoted by the root dacry-. Some illustrations will make the distinction clearer:

dacryoadenitis (dacry/o/aden/itis) — inflammation of a lacrimal gland (a tear gland)
dacryocystectomy (dacry/o/cyst/ectomy) — excision of the wall of the lacrimal sac

Note the relationships:

tear gland = lacrimal gland = dacryadeno-
tear sac (or bladder) = lacrimal sac = dacrycysto-

dura   hard / used principally as a shortened form of dura mater, the outermost, toughest and most fibrous of the three membranes (meninges) covering the brain and spinal cord

Examples:

dura mater (or dura) — the outermost of the three membranes covering the brain and spinal cord
induration (in/dur/ation) — hardness; the act or process of becoming hard (**in-** has the ordinary sense of "within," thus induration has the literal meaning of "a process of within or inner hardness")
superdural (super/dur/al) — situated above or external to the dura mater

fascia   sheet; band / a sheet or band of fibrous tissue

The name fascia is used to denote connective tissues which exist extensively throughout the body and serve the purpose of forming an outer layer for other tissues such as ligaments and tendons; fascia also serve as anchors or binders to support or hold other tissue structures such as muscle bundles which are held together and kept in place during movement by a sheathlike covering of fascia

Examples:

fasciculus (fasci/cul/us) — a small bundle or cluster; used to designate a small bundle of nerve or muscle fibers
fasciodesis (fasci/o/desis) — the operation of suturing a fascia to one of the tissues attached to the skeleton
fasciorrhaphy (fasci/o/rrhaphy) — the suturing together of torn fascia

Lesson 7 — Reading Assignment

helio-   sun; light / sunlight

This root is used principally to designate effects of the rays of the sun as in:
   heliosensitivity (helio/sensitivity) — sensitivity to sunlight
   heliosis (helio/sis) — sunstroke
   heliotherapy (helio/therapy) — the treatment of disease by exposing the body to the sun's rays; therapeutic sunbathing

hypno-   sleep

Examples:
   hypnotic (hypnot/ic) — inducing sleep; a drug that acts to induce sleep; pertaining to or of the nature of hypnotism
   hypnotism (hypnot/ism) — the method or practice of an artificially induced passive state in which there is increased responsiveness to suggestions and commands
   ahypnia (a/hypn/ia) — "not sleep" (You will recall that the prefix **a-** has a meaning "not."); abnormal wakefulness; insomnia

iso-   equal / alike; the same

This prefix is used widely to indicate "sameness' as in:
   isocellular (iso/cell/ul/ar) — composed of cells of the same size and kind
   isopia (is/op/ia) — equality of vision in the two eyes

The prefix **iso-** can also be combined with the prefix **an-** meaning "not," to indicate "not equal" or "inequality."
   anisodont (an/is/odont) — having teeth of unequal size or length
   anisopia (an/is/op/ia) — inequality of vision in the two eyes
   anisomastia (an/iso/mast/ia) — inequality of the breasts

lapar-   abdominal wall / loin (the part of the back between the end of the ribs and the hip), flank (the part of the side between the ribs and the hip)

Technically the root **lapar-** applies to the lower back and sides, that is, the soft fleshy parts of the back and sides between the bones of the ribs and the hip bone. However, the root is used loosely to include the front of the cavity as well. It is in this looser or wider sense that the frequent word laparotomy is used.
   laparotomy (lapar/otomy) — surgical incision of the flank; less correctly but more generally, abdominal incision at any point in the abdominal wall

Examples:
   hysterolaparotomy (hyster/o/lapar/otomy) — incision of the womb through the abdominal wall
   thoracolaparotomy (thorac/o/lapar/otomy) — incision through both the thorax and the abdomen
   laparorrhaphy (lapar/o/rrhaphy) — suturing of the abdominal wall
   laparogastrostomy (lapar/o/gastr/ostomy) — the creation of a permanent opening to the stomach through the abdominal wall

malign-   bad; harmful

Examples:
   malignant (malign/ant) — tending to become progressively worse and to result in death
   malignancy (malign/ancy) — a tendency to spread or become progressively worse; used most frequently with cancerous growths which tend to progressively invade (spread among) the tissues of the body

Malignant and benign (lesson 4) are opposites.

Lesson 7 — Reading Assignment

ment-   the mind

Examples:
mental (ment/al) — pertaining to the mind
mentality (ment/al/ity) — mental power or activity
dementia (de/ment/ia) — a general term for mental deterioration (the prefix **de-** means "down," "down from")

The root **ment-** meaning "mind" is not extensively used in forming medical terms, the root **psych-** being the preferred element in words or expressions relating to the mind. Also, there may be confusion with the more widely used root ment- meaning "chin."

ocul-   eye

Examples:
ocular (ocul/ar) — pertaining to the eye
oculus (ocul/us) — name for the eye

In Lesson 2 we learned the roots **ophthalm-** and **opt-** which also have to do with vision and sight. Following is a comparison of the various roots having to do with the eye:
ocul-   form denoting relationship to the eye
ophthalm-   form denoting relationship to the eye
opt-   form meaning visible, or denoting relationship to vision or sight
-opia (-op/ia) — suffix element denoting a condition of vision or sight

opt- and -opia related to the function of the eye, that is vision or seeing

ocul- and ophthalm- relate to the eye as a physical or anatomical organ

ocul-   is generally used as a landmark
ophthalm-   is generally used to designate conditions of the eye and therapy applied to the eye

Examples:
oculonasal (ocul/o/nas/al) — pertaining to the eye and the nose
oculopathy (ocul/o/path/y) — any disease or disorder of the eye

part-   labor; bring forth / bear / giving birth; delivery

This root is closely related to our common use of the word **part** in the sense of "to separate from" since delivery or giving birth is the process whereby the mother is separated or "parted" from her offspring.

Examples:
parturition (part/ur/ition) — the act or process of giving birth to a child
postpartum (post/part/um) — occurring after childbirth or after delivery
  post- means "after" and is discussed more fully in Lesson 10)
prepartal (pre/part/al) — occurring before or just previous to labor
  pre- means "before" and is discussed more fully in Lesson 10)

pod-   foot

Examples:
podalic (pod/al/ic) — accomplished by means of the foot, as in obstetrical deliveries (versions)
-podia (-pod/ia) — condition of the foot

102

Lesson 7 — Reading Assignment

There is a related root **ped-** which may denote either foot or child:

pedodontics (ped/odont/ics) — the department of dentistry dealing with the oral health of children

pedopathy (ped/o/path/y) — any disease of the foot

pediatrician (ped/iatr/ician) — a physician specializing in the diseases of children

Examples:

podiatry (pod/iatr/y) — the diagnosis and treatment of diseases of the foot

podiatrist (pod/iatr/ist) — one who practices podiatry. Usually, a podiatrist is not a doctor of medicine and is limited by his license to diseases of the foot

scirr(h)-   hard / relating to a hard tumor

The root scirr- (frequently scirrh-) is used to denote relationships to a scirrhus which is the name for a hard, cancerous tumor.

Examples:

scirrhus (scirrh/us) — name for a hard, cancerous tumor

scirrhous (scirrh/ous) — pertaining to or of the nature of a scirrhus

-scirrhus is also used as a word ending, the first element(s) in the word adding additional description:

mastoscirrhus (mast/o/scirrh/us) — a hard cancer of the breast

dacryadenoscirrhus (dacry/aden/o/scirrh/us) — a hard cancerous tumor (a scirrhus) of the lacrimal (tear) gland

scler(a)   hard / hardness; also "the white of the eye"

Since the presence of hardness in body parts which are normally lacking in hardness is a frequent sign of a morbid (diseased) condition, the root scler- is widely used in medical terms to indicate the condition of abnormal hardness.

sclerous (scler/ous) — hard; indurated (in/dur/ated)

sclerosis (scler/osis) — a hardening; an induration; especially hardening of a part from inflammation. May also be used as a word ending (-sclerosis) with preceeding element(s) in the word providing more information.

Another frequent use of the element scler- is in reference to the sclera, "the white of the eye," the white cover of the eyeball which surrounds the back five-sixths of the eyeball. (The front one-sixth of this cover is called the cornea and will be discussed in Lesson 8.)

sclera (scler/a) — the tough, white supporting cover of the eyeball covering approximately the back five-sixths of its surface

sclerotic (sclerot/ic) — pertaining to hardness or hardening; pertaining to the sclera

Usages of **dura, scirrh-, scler-**:

In this lesson we have presented three elements all of which carry a meaning of "hardness." Following is a clarifying summary:

dura is used principally as a shortened name for the **dura mater**, the hard outer covering of the brain and spinal cord. An important exception to this usage is the word induration (in/dur/ation) which means "hardness or "the process of hardening."

scirrh- is used almost exclusively in reference to a hard, cancerous tumor.

scler- can mean "hardness or be a reference to "the white of the eye."

Lesson 7 — Reading Assignment

sept-   wall; fence / a dividing wall or membrane

Examples:
septum (sept/um) — a general term in anatomy to designate a dividing wall or partition
nasal septum (nas/al sept/um) — the partition separating the two nasal cavities (nostrils).
   When sept- is used with no other qualification as in septectomy (sept/ectomy), septotomy
   (sept/otomy), the reference is to the nasal septum.
septal (sept/al) — pertaining to a septum
septulum (sept/ul/um) — a small separating wall or partition

sinus   hollow space / cavity; hollow; recess

There are many cavities, hollows and spaces in the body which are designated as sinuses. The
most familiar are the para/nasal sinuses which are air cavities in the cranial bones communicating
with the nasal cavity.

Examples:
sinusoid (sinus/oid) — resembling a sinus; used to designate blood channels in organs such as
   the heart, liver, spleen, pancreas
sinusotomy (sinus/otomy) — surgical incision of a sinus
sinusology (sinus/ology) — that branch of medicine which has to do with the sinuses

somato-   body / the body

Examples:
somal, somatic (som/al, somat/ic) — pertaining to the body
soma (som/a) — denoting the body as distinguished from the mind

The elements som-, somat- are used to refer to the body as a whole, as in:
somatomegaly (somat/o/megal/y) — abnormal size of a body; giantism
somatotherapy (somat/o/therap/y) — treatment aimed at curing the ills of the body
somasthenia (som/asthenia) — a condition of bodily weakness

Or, the elements may be used to emphasize the body as distinct from the mind, as in:
somatopathy (somat/o/path/y) — a bodily disorder as distinguished from a mental one
somatopsychic (somat/o/psych/ic) — pertaining to both body and mind
psychosomatic (psych/o/somat/ic) — pertaining to the mind-body relationship; having bodily
   symptoms of a psychic, emotional or mental origin

tarso-   ankle region; instep

Examples:
tarsus (tars/us) — the ankle region
tarsal (tars/al) — pertaining to the instep; pertaining to the ankle bones (tarsal bones)
metatarsus (meta/tars/us) — the part of the foot between the ankle (tarsus) and the toes. (Meta-
   means "beyond," therefore, the literal translation of metatarsus is "beyond the tarsus," "beyond the ankle")
metatarsal (meta/tars/al) — pertaining to the metatarsus; one of the five bones between the
   ankle and the toes

-tope   place / location

The chief application of this suffix is in the word *isotope* which denotes forms of a chemical
element which have identical chemical properties but different atomic weights. So called because
they are put in the "same place" in the Periodic Table (classification of elements).

Lesson 7 — Reading Assignment

A much wider use is made of the root *top-* meaning "place," "locality," or "local."

-ectopia (-ec/top/ia) — a suffix meaning displacement; literally, "a condition of (ia) out of (ec-) place (top)." The stem is attached to organs or parts indicating such a displacement: oste/o/ec/topia, my/ec/top/ia.

The element may have the meaning of "local" or "localized" as opposed to "general" or "widespread."

topical (top/ic/al) — pertaining to a particular spot; local; as in topical anesthesia (local anesthesia) versus general anesthesia

topalgia (top/algia) — fixed or localized pain

trachel-   neck or necklike structure

Trachel- applies to a neck or necklike structure and is most frequently used with reference to the neck of the body or the neck (cervix) of the uterus (womb).

Another root closely resembling trachel- is the element *trache-* which refers to the windpipe, the main trunk of the system of tubes by which air passes to and from the lungs.

trachea (trache/a) — name of the windpipe
tracheal (trache/al) — pertaining to the windpipe

Following is a review of the elements denoting a neck or necklike structure which are used interchangeably:

cervic/o-, trachel/o-   combining forms indicating relationship to a neck or necklike structure

cervic/itis, trachel/itis — inflammation of the uterine cervic (neck of the womb)

(Note: trache/itis is inflammation of the trachea the windpipe)

Examples:
trachelocystitis (trachel/o/cyst/itis) — inflammation of the neck of the bladder
trachelodynia (trachel/odyn/ia) — pain in the neck
trachelomyitis (trachel/o/my/itis) — inflammation of the muscles of the neck

Lesson 7 — Element Recognition Exercise

Separate the elements, connecting vowels, and word terminals of the following medical words by inserting a slash mark (/) between them.

Example: trachelocystitis — trachel/o/cyst/itis

heliopathia

astrocytoma

leiasthenia

fasciodesis

isogenesis

tarsomegaly

topalgia

podarthritis

malignant

adnexogenesis

oculopathy

laparocholecystotomy

dacryocystorhinostenosis

scleradenitis

somatasthenia

trachelodynia

sinusotomy

hypnogenic

scirrhoblepharoncus

antrostomy

endocrinopathy

adnexectomy

laparosalpingotomy

dacryoadenalgia

sclerostenosis

somatesthesia

trachelomyitis

sinusitis

hypnalgia

antrectomy

crinogenic

heliosis

astrocyte

gastrasthenia

fasciorrhaphy

isocytosis

tarsoptosis

topesthesia

pododynia

dacryolithiasis

somatopsychic

sinusoid

Lesson 8 — Review

ELEMENT	AUDIONYM	VISUAL IMAGE	MEANING
pneum-	name	See the **name** plate turned into a **lung**!	lung, air
phage	page	See the **page eat**ing!	to eat
phren-	friend	See the people pulling on the **frien**d saying, **"mine! mine! mine!"**!	mind
corne-	corn	See the **corn** with **horn**s growing out of it!	horny, hornlike
plak-	plaque	See the **plaque** with a **plate** of food on it!	plate
iris	I race	See the person saying, **"I race"** while racing up the **rainbow**!	rainbow (eye membrane)
kerat-	carrot	See the **carrot** with **horns** growing out of it!	horny, horny tissue
pulmon- pulmo-	pull moon	See someone **pul**ling on the **mo**on and the moon is a **lung**!	lung
ptyal-	tile	See the **tile** with a **sail**boat on it!	saliva
alveol-	owl field	See the **owl** in the **field** falling into a **cave-in** (cavity)!	cavity, socket
oophor-	over	See the **over**turned **egg** and **eggs** being turned **over**!	ovary (one of two female reproductive glands)
oment-	"O" men	See the **"O" men** with the **covering** over their heads!	covering (of internal abdominal organs)
sedat-	seated	See the speaker saying, "Be **seated**" and the audience becoming **quiet** and **calm**!	quiet, calm

Lesson 8 — Review

ELEMENT	AUDIONYM	VISUAL IMAGE	MEANING
furca-	fur coat	See the **fur co**at covered with **fork**s!	fork-shaped
radic-	radish	See the **radi**sh with the **root** beer bursting out of it!	root
radi-	radio	See the **radi**o with a **ray** beaming out of it!	ray
fistul-	fist	See the **fist** full of **pipes**!	pipe, a narrow passage
edema-	a demon	See **a dem**on **swelling** and **swelling**!	swelling (by fluid)
dactyl-	duck tail	See the **duck tail** with a **finger** and **toe** growing out of it!	finger, toe
metabol(e)	met a bull	See the man who **met a bul**l asking it for **change**!	change
pariet-	parrot	See the **parrot** with **walls** on its sides!	wall
ependym-	a pendulum	See **a pendu**lum with **wrapping** all over it!	wrapping, a covering
gravid	gravity	See the image for **gravi**ty, a **pra**ying **nut** falling from a tree!	pregnant
aer-	air (plane)	See the **air**plane with **air** coming out of it in all directions!	air
glyco- gluco-	glide coal	See the **gli**ding **co**al with **Sweet** Chocolate for wings!	sweet, sugar

Lesson 8 — Worksheet

Complete the following:

ELEMENT	AUDIONYM	MEANING
pneum-		
phage		
phren-		
corne-		
plak-		
iris		
kerat-		
pulmon- pulmo-		
ptyal-		
alveol-		
oophor-		
oment-		
sedat-		
furca-		
radic-		
radi-		
fistul-		
edema-		
dactyl-		
metabol(e)		
pariet-		
ependym-		
gravid		
aer-		
glyco- gluco-		

Lesson 8 — Word Terminals

-ization   action or process

This terminal is a combination of **-ize** and **-ation.**

 -ize   to do, to act in a specified way

Examples:

 liquid/ize, union/ize, critic/ize, brutal/ize

 -ation   (see Word Terminals, Lesson 4) a process, action or condition

Examples:

 commercial/ization, real/ization, crystall/ization

-ity   condition; character

Examples:

 formal/ity, normal/ity, civil/ity

-ive   of, relating to, having the nature or quality of

Examples:

 nat/ive, substant/ive, sedat/ive, direct/ive

-or   a person or thing that does something or has some particular function

In Lesson 4 the terminal **-or** was defined as "that which does something or has some particular function." All we are doing here is including "a person or thing" as one of the "that which does."

Examples:

 invent/or, object/or, elevat/or, sail/or, vend/or

-ence   is another form of **-ance** (Word Terminals, Lesson 7) and means the same thing, that is, "a state or condition; the act of"

Lesson 8 — Reading Assignment

aer-   air / gas

This element represents an older spelling of air and persists in medical terminology. It is used to indicate air or an otherwise unspecified gas.

Examples:
  aerial (aer/i/al) — pertaining to the air
  aerosis (aer/osis) — the production of gas in the tissues or organs of the body
  aeropathy (aer/o/path/y) — any disease due to a change in atmospheric pressure such as compressed air illness ("bends") or air sickness

alveol-   cavity; socket / small cavity, pit or hollow

This root is used most frequently in reference to the cavities or sockets of either jaw in which the roots of the teeth are embedded. (Note: Cavity as used here is a hollow space and does not refer to the pits in the teeth resulting from decay which are more properly dental caries.)

Examples:
  alveolus (alveol/us) — (plural alveoli) name used to designate a small saclike pit or cavity
  dental alveoli (dent/al alveol/i) — the tooth sockets in the upper and lower jaw bones
  alveolar (alveol/ar) — pertaining to an alveolus
  alveolectomy (alveol/ectomy) — surgical excision of the tooth socket bony structure as a preparatory measure for the wearing of false teeth (dent/ures); may include the removal of remaining teeth and roots of teeth and excision of diseased tissue
  alveoloplasty (alveol/o/plast/y) — the surgical improvement of the shape and condition of the tooth sockets in preparation for immediate or future denture construction

corne-   horny, hornlike / the cornea of the eye, the transparent part of the covering of the eyeball which covers the iris and pupil and admits light to the interior

Examples:
  corn — the name of a build-up of thick horny skin tissue produced by friction and pressure
  corneal (corne/al) — pertaining to the cornea of the eye
  corneous (corne/ous) — hornlike or horny

dactyl-   finger; toe / digit (Note: a digit is a finger or a toe; a finger is a "digit of the hand," a toe is a "digit of the foot.")

Examples:
  dactyloscopy (dactyl/o/scop/y) — examination of fingerprints for purpose of identification
  -dactylia, sometimes -dactyly (-dactyl/ia, -dactyl/y) — a condition of the fingers or toes

Note: In medical terminology the fingers and toes are technically called digits; although the element dactyl- applies to fingers and toes, it is more frequently used for the fingers.

Examples:
  isodactylisrn (iso/dactyl/ism) — a condition in which the fingers are of relatively equal length
  dactylospasm (dactyl/o/spasm) — a spasm or cramp of a finger or toe

-edema   swelling by fluid) / an abnormal accumulation of fluid in cells, tissues or cavities of the body, resulting in swelling

Example:
  edematous (edemat/ous) — pertaining to or affected by edema

Lesson 8 — Reading Assignment

Edema can be used as a word to form terms such as "edema of_____" or as a suffix to indicate the location or the kind of fluid accumulation:

pneumonedema (pneumon/edema) — abnormal quantities of fluid in the lungs
dactyledema (dactyl/edema) — abnormal swelling of the fingers or toes due to fluid accumulation

ependym-   wrapping; a covering / specifically, the membrane lining the cavities of the brain and the canal enclosing the spinal cord

Examples:
ependyma (ependym/a) — name of the membrane lining the cavities of the brain and the canal enclosing the spinal cord
ependymal (ependym/al) — pertaining to or composed of ependyma
ependymopathy (ependym/o/path/y) — any disease of this membrane (the ependyma)
ependymitis (ependym/itis) — inflammation of the ependyma

fistul-   pipe; a narrow passage / an abnormal passage leading from an abscess (a collection of pus in a cavity) or hollow organ to the body surface, or from one hollow organ to another and permitting passage of fluids (as pus) or secretions (as saliva)

Examples:
fistula (fistul/a) — term for such an abnormal passage
fistulous (fistul/ous) — pertaining to or of the nature of a fistula

Fistulas are described by their location:

internal fistula — an abnormal passage between two internal organs
external fistula — an abnormal passage between a hollow organ and the external surface of the body
intestinal fistula — an abnormal passage connecting with the intestine

Sometimes a fistula may be surgically created as a therapeutic measure:

fistulization (fistul/ization) — the process of becoming fistulous; the surgical creation of an opening into a hollow organ or of an opening between two structures which were not previously connected
fistuloenterostomy (fistul/o/enter/ostomy) — the operation of making a fistula empty permanently into the intestine

furca-   fork-shaped / frequently used to designate the area between the roots of the teeth

Examples:
furcal (furc/al) — shaped like a fork; forked
bifurcate (bi/furc/ate) — forked; divided into two like a fork (***bi-*** means "two" and is discussed more fully in Lesson 12)
bifurcation (bi/furc/ation) — division into two branches; the site where a single structure divides into two

glyco-, gluco-   sweet; sugary / sugar

This root is chiefly used to indicate the presence of sugar in the blood:

glycemia (glyc/em/ia) — the presence of sugar in the blood
hyperglycemia (hyper/glyc/em/ia) — abnormally increased content of sugar in the blood

Lesson 8 — Reading Assignment

Examples:

glycolysis (glyc/o/lysis) — the breaking down of sugar into simpler compounds

glycopenia (glyc/o/penia) — a deficiency of sugar in the body tissues

glucose (gluc/ose) — a thick, syrupy, sweet liquid; the sweet, colorless, soluble form of dextrose that occurs widely in nature and is the usual form in which carbohydrate is assimilated by animals

gravid   pregnant

Examples:

gravid — pregnant; containing developing young

gravidic (gravid/ic) — occurring during pregnancy

gravidity (gravid/ity) — the condition of being with child; pregnancy

gravidocardiac (gravid/o/cardi/ac) — pertaining to heart disease of pregnancy

iris   rainbow (eye membrane) / specifically, the colored membrane of the eye

Examples:

iris — name of the colored membrane of the eye

iridic, sometimes iridal (irid/ic, irid/al) — pertaining to the iris

iridization (irid/iz/ation) — the patient's perception of colored halos about lights, occurring in glaucoma (a disease of the eye marked by increased pressure within the eyeball)

kerat-   horny; horny tissue / also the cornea of the eye

Examples:

keratic (kerat/ic) — pertaining to horny tissue; pertaining to the cornea

keratoderma (kerat/o/derma) — a horny skin or covering

keratoid (kerat/oid) — resembling horny or corneal tissue

hyperkeratosis (hyper/kerat/osis — overgrowth (excessive growth) of the horny layer of the skin

keratomalacia (kerat/o/malacia) — softening of the cornea

keratocentesis (kerat/o/centesis) — puncture of the cornea

Comparison between kerat/o- and corne-:

corne-   is used principally to designate the cornea of the eye as a structure and landmark

kerat/o-   is used to designate horny tissues and conditions and therapeutic procedures related to the cornea

metabol(e)   change

Examples:

metabolism (metabol/ism) — the sum of all the physical and chemical processes by which living organized substance is produced and maintained, and also the transformation by which energy is made available for the use of the body

basal metabolism — the minimal energy needed to maintain the physical and chemical activities of the body

oment-   covering (of internal abdominal organs) / the membrane in the front part of the abdomen which folds over and supports the stomach, liver and parts of the intestine

Examples:

omentum (oment/um) — name of the membranous cover of the abdominal organs

omental (oment/al) — pertaining to the omentum

omentopexy (oment/o/pexy) — the attachment of the omentum to another tissue or organ

Lesson 8 — Reading Assignment

omentoplasty (oment/o/plast/y) — the use of omental grafts, that is, surgical repair using the omentum as the grafting material

oophor- ovary / literally "egg carrier" (oo-, egg or ovum + phor-, carrier); either of the pair of female reproductive glands producing eggs and sex hormones

As is indicated above the elements **oophor-** and **ovar-** are synonyms, ovar- being more frequently used to designate the anatomical part and oophor- being more frequently used to name diseases, abnormalities and therapeutic procedures applied to these reproductive glands.

Examples:
oophoron (oophor/on) — an ovary

oophoropexy (oophor/o/pexy) — the surgical fixation or attaching of the ovary (also called adnex/o/pexy; You will recall that an adnexus is an appendage or attachment. The ovaries [oophor-] the uterine tubes [salping-], and the ligaments are considered as appendages of the uterus [uterine adnexa].)

hystero-oophorectomy (hyster/o/oophor/ectomy) — surgical removal (excision) of the uterus and ovaries (also called oophor/o/hyster/ectomy)

pariet- wall / wall of an organ or cavity

This element may be used to denote a wall or a side of an organ or cavity of the body. It is used chiefly to designate two bones which form the side walls of the cranium, the parietal bones.

Example:
parietal (pariet/al) — pertaining to the walls of a cavity

phage to eat / eating, swallowing

Examples:
onychophagy (onych/o/phag/y) — nail biting

phagomania (phag/o/mani/a) — an insatiable craving for food; literally an "eating mania"

phagocyte (phag/o/cyt/e) — any cell that absorbs ("eats") micro-organisms, other cells, and foreign bodies

phagocytosis (phag/o/cyt/osis) — the process of engulfing a micro-organism, other cells and foreign bodies by phagocytes

odynophagia (odyn/o/phag/ia) — pain in swallowing

phren- mind / also the diaphragm; also the phrenic nerve, a nerve with branches spreading mostly over the lower part of the diaphragm

The diaphragm is the muscular wall or partition separating the chest cavity and the abdominal cavity; the "midriff."

Examples:
phrenic (phren/ic) — pertaining to the mind; pertaining to the diaphragm

phrenic- (phren/ic-) — form denoting relationship to the phrenic nerve

The suffix -phrenia is used to form words having to do with mental disorders:

bradyphrenia (brady/phren/ia) — slowness of mental activity such as initiative, interest, speech, frequently accompanying encephalitis

Note: The ancient Greeks, from whose language this root is taken, believed that the diaphragm was the location of the mind just as we, today, believe that the head (actually the brain) is the

Lesson 8 — Reading Assignment

location of the mind. It would have been as commonplace for the Greeks to describe a person as having a good "diaphragm" as for us to describe a person as having a good "head"; both usages would indicate a good "mind."

plak-   a plate / also plaque; a patch of eruption

This root appears in the form -plak/ia and indicates a forming of patches of eruption, usually on mucous membrane:

    leukoplakia (leuk/o/plak/ia) — a disease marked by white thickened patches on the mucous membrane of the cheeks, gum and tongue
    malacoplakia (malac/o/plak/ia) — the formation of soft patches on the mucous membrane of a hollow organ

  plaque — any patch or flat area

    dental plaque — a deposit of material on the surface of a tooth

pneum-   the lungs; air

The importance of air to maintain life is reflected in the various forms in which the element **pne-** is applied in the formation of medical terms. The presence of the root **pne-** in a word indicates a relationship to air or breathing.

  -pnea (-pne/a) — breathing

    hyperpnea (hyper/pne/a) — abnormal increase in the speed and depth of breathing
    hypopnea (hypo/pne/a) — abnormal decrease in the speed and depth of breathing
    bradypnea (brady/pne/a) — abnormal slowness of breathing

  pneum-, pneumat-   forms indicating a relationship to air or to respiration (the inhalation and exhalation of air)

    pneumal (pneum/al) — pertaining to the lungs
    pneumatic (pneumat/ic) — of or pertaining to air or respiration
    pneumatocele (pneumat/o/cele) — a swelling containing air any place in the body; a pushing out of the lung through a weak place in the wall of the chest

  pneumon-   form indicating a relationship to the lungs

    pneumonia (pneumon/ia) — inflammation of the lungs, usually with complications and usually accompanied by chill, increase in temperature, pain and coughing
    pneumonitis (pneumon/itis) — a condition of localized, acute inflammation of the lung without the range of complications and symptoms accompanying pneumonia; benign pneumonia
    pneumonic (pneumon/ic) — pertaining to the lung or to pneumonia

ptyal-   saliva / spit

Examples:
    ptyalism (ptyal/ism) — excessive secretion of saliva; salivation
    -ptysis (-pty/sis) — the spitting of —

      hemoptysis (hem/o/pty/sis) — the spitting of blood or of blood stained spittle (sputum)

    ptyalectasis (ptyal/ectasis) — dilatation (enlarging) of a salivary duct by surgery
    ptyalogenic (ptyal/o/gen/ic) — formed from or by the action of saliva

Lesson 8 — Reading Assignment

pulmon-   lung

Examples:
pulmo (pulm/o) — the lung, the organ of respiration
pulmonic, pulmonary (pulmon/ic, pulmon/ary) — pertaining to the lungs

-pulmonary (-pulmon/ary) is used as a suffix denoting relationship to the lungs and the preceding element

renopulmonary (ren/o/pulmon/ary) — pertaining to the kidney and lungs

Comparison of *pulm/o*, *pulmon/o-* with *pneumon/o*:

pulm/o- and pulmon/o-   are used, principally, to indicate the lung as a landmark

pneumon/o-   is used principally to name conditions and therapeutic procedures applied to the lungs

radi-   ray; beam; spoke

This root is used to convey the idea of something which spreads out from the center like spokes from the hub of a wheel; it is used particularly in medicine to denote the process whereby energy in the form of light, heat and X-rays is emitted.

Examples:
radial (radi/al) — pertaining to rays; pertaining to the spreading out from the center
radiology (radi/ology) — the study of X-rays, frequently called roentgenology after Wilhelm Konrad Roentgen, the discoverer of X-rays
radiotherapy (radi/o/therap/y) — the treatment of disease by the use of X-rays or rays from a radioactive substance

radic-   root / origin

Examples:
radical (radic/al) — directed to the cause; going to the root or source of a morbid process
radix — "the root"; the lowermost part, or a structure by which something is firmly attached
radicle (radi/cle) — "a little root"; any one of the smallest branches of a vessel or nerve

The form radicul- (radic/ul-) usually denotes a nerve root, particularly the spinal nerve roots:

radiculectomy (radic/ul/ectomy) — excision of a nerve root
radiculoneuropathy (radic/ul/o/neur/o/path/y) — disease of the nerve roots and the nerve *(neur-* is a root meaning "nerve" and is discussed more fully in Lesson 10)

sedat-   quiet; calm

Examples:
sedation (sedat/ion) — the act or process of calming
sedative (sedat/ive) — an agent such as a drug that calms or reduces excitement

Lesson 8 — Element Recognition Exercise

Separate the elements, connecting vowels, and word terminals of the following medical words by inserting a slash mark (/) between them.

Example: oophorocystectomy — oophor/o/cyst/ectomy

pneumomelanosis

phagocytolysis

phrenasthenia

iridectasis

keratogenesis

pulmonitis

ptyalolithiasis

alveolodontal

oophorohysterectomy

omentorrhaphy

sedative

furcal

radiectomy

radiocarcinogenesis

fistulectomy

cephaledema

dactylospasm

metabology

parietitis

ependymitis

gravidocardiac

aerenterectasia

hyperglycodermia

alveolalgia

omentitis

radical

dactylogram

metabolism

ependymocyte

aerendocardia

glycopenia

pneumohypoderma

phagomania

phrenitis

iridoptosis

keratoderma

pulmonectomy

ptyalogenic

phrenopathy

keratoma

ptyalolithotomy

ependyma

Lesson 9 — Review

ELEMENT	AUDIONYM	VISUAL IMAGE	MEANING
tarso-	tar	See the **tar** with triangles stuck into it and the **framework of the upper eyelid** attached to it!	framework of the upper eyelid
cheir- chir-	care (package)	See the **Care** Package with a **hand** sticking out of it!	hand
calc-	calculator	See the **calc**ulator with a **heel** and a **stone** on top of it!	heel, stone
cine-	Sen Sen	See the **Sen Sen** (mints) **moving** on their own!	move, movement
digit	dig it	See the shovel (**dig it**) with a **finger** and **toe** on it!	finger, toe
dors-	doors	See the double **do**ors with a **back** on each of them!	back
gangli-	gang	See the **gang** robbing the bank. The **gang** is **swelling** and **swelling**!	swelling, knotlike mass
gemin-	gem	See the **gem**s. They are **twins**, they are **doubles**!	twin, double
grad-	graduate	See the **grad**uate **walk** away and **take** the **steps**!	walk, take steps
gran-	grandma	See **gran**dma eating **grain particles**!	grain, particle
labi-	lab	See the test tube (**lab**) with **lips** on it!	lip
micr-	microphone	See the **micr**ophone so **small** that it is no higher than the speaker's toe!	small

118

Lesson 9— Review

ELEMENT	AUDIONYM	VISUAL IMAGE	MEANING
peps- pept-	Pepsi	See the **Peps**i bottle with the Readers **Digest** stuck into it!	digest
pleur-	pliers	See the **plier**s with **rib**s on its **side**s!	pleura (membrane) rib, side
mamm-	mammal	See the whale (**mamm**al) with a **breast!**	breast
colla-	cola	See the **Cola** bottle with **glue** in it!	glue, gelatin like
later-	ladder	See the **lad**der with the person climbing up the **side** of it!	side
rachi-	rake	See the **rake** made of a **spinal column**!	spinal column
phob-	foe	See the **foe** whose shield is made of **fur**!	fear
phot-	photo	See the **phot**o with a **light** shining out of it!	light
dys-	dice	See the **dice** with a **bat** stuck through them!	bad, out of order
cut-	cut	See the image for "**cut**," scissors made of **skin**!	skin
en-	hen	See the h**en** saying, "They won't let me **in** the **Inn**"!	in
peri-	pear	See the **pear** having **a bout** with **a round** pear!	about, around
pro-	pro	See the **pro** golfer with the people walking **in front of** the ball **before** the **pro** can hit it!	in front of, before

119

Lesson 9 — Worksheet

Complete the following:

ELEMENT	AUDIONYM	MEANING
tarso-		
cheir- chir-		
calc-		
cine-		
digit		
dors-		
gangli-		
gemin-		
grad-		
gran-		
labi-		
micr-		
peps- pept-		
pleur-		
mamm-		
colla-		
later-		
rachi-		
phob-		
phot-		
dys-		
cut-		
en-		
peri-		
pro-		

Lesson 9 — Reading Assignment

calc-   heel; stone / basically refers to calcium, one of the essential materials in the body

This element may appear as calc- referring to the element calcium:

   calcic (calc/ic) — of, or pertaining to, calcium
   calcemia (calc/em/ia) — the presence of an abnormally large amount of calcium in the blood

Or, it may appear as calcan- referring to the heel bone:

   calcaneus (calcane/us) — name of the heel bone, the large tarsal (ankle) bone which forms the heel

Or, it may appear as calcare- referring to the various chemical compounds containing calcium; lime and chalky substances are chemical forms containing calcium:

   calcareous (calcare/ous) — pertaining to or containing lime or calcium; chalky

cheir-, chir-   hand

   Examples:
   chiropractic (chir/o/pract/ic) — a method of treating disease by manipulation of the body, especially manipulation of the spine with the hands
   chiropractor (chir/o/pract/or) — one who practices chiropractic
   cheirarthritis (cheir/arthr/itis) — inflammation of the joints of the hands including the joints of the fingers

cine-   move; movement / also kine-

The form cine- is used principally to refer to the use of photographic or motion picture techniques in studying motion in the various organs such as the heart.
   cineradiography (cine/radi/o/graph/y) — the making of motion pictures of images produced by X-rays
   cineangiography (cine/angi/o/graph/y) — the recording of the images of the blood vessels through motion picture techniques

The form kine- is used to denote the more general relationship to movement:

   kine-, kinesi- (kine/si-) — forms denoting relationship to movement
   kinemia (kin/em/ia) — movement of the blood from the heart
   kinesitherapy (kines/i/therap/y) — the treatment of disease by movements or exercise
   -kinesia, -kinesis (-kines/ia, -kine/sis) — combinations meaning abnormal movement
   bradykinesia (brady/kines/ia) — slow movement

Another form, kinet-, is used with the meaning "movable "

   kinet-   form meaning "movable"
   kinetic (kinet/ic) — pertaining to or producing motion
   kinetism (kinet/ism) — the ability to perform or begin muscular motion

colla   glue; gelatinlike; starch

   Examples:
   collagen (colla/gen) — the gelatinlike or sticky substance of skin, bone, cartilage and connective tissue
   collagenous (colla/gen/ous) — forming or producing collagen; pertaining to collagen

Lesson 9 — Reading Assignment

collagenogenic (colla/gen/o/gen/ic) — pertaining to the production of collagen
colloid (coll/oid) — gelatinlike or resembling glue or starch

cut-   skin

Examples:
cutis (cut/is) — the skin; the outer protective covering of the body
cuticle (cut/icle) — "a little skin"; the outer layer of the skin; the ep/onych/ium
cutaneous (cutan/eous) — pertaining to the skin
-cutaneous (-cutan/eous) — suffix denoting relationship to the skin

subcutaneous (sub/cutan/eous) — situated or occurring beneath the skin
transcutaneous (trans/cutan/eous) — through the skin

cutitis (cut/itis) — inflammation of the skin

digit   finger; toe / medical word used to name a finger or a toe

Example:
digital (digit/al) — pertaining to the digits (fingers or toes)
(See discussion of dactyl — Lesson 8)

dors-   back / the back of the body; the body as viewed from the back

This root is used principally to denote the back of the body or the back of any body part as a landmark; the meaning would be close to "back side."

Examples:
dorsum (dors/um) — name for the back; the back of the body
dorsal (dors/al) — pertaining to the back or the "back side"; denoting a position more toward the back surface than to some other object of reference
dorsad (dors/ad) — toward the back or the "back side"
subdorsal (sub/dors/al) — situated below the dorsal (back) region
dorsolateral (dors/o/later/al) — pertaining to the back and side

dys-   bad; out of order / difficult; painful; opposite of "good"

Examples:
dysentery (dys/enter/y) — abdominal disorders marked by inflammation of the intestines and accompanied by pain in the abdomen, cramp and frequent bowel movements containing blood and mucus
dyspepsia (dys/peps/ia) — indigestion; a weakening or lessening of the power or function of digestion
dysphagia (dys/phag/ia) — difficulty in swallowing
dyspnea (dys/pne/a) — difficult or labored breathing
dystrophy (dys/trophy) — a disorder arising from defective or faulty nutrition; faulty development

en-   in / within; inside; usually em- before b, m, or p

Examples:
empathy (em/path/y) — "feeling within"; the entering into the feelings of another person
encephal- (en/cephal-) — "within the head"; usually with reference to the brain; however, the reference may be to other conditions within the head as, for example, encephalalgia, "pain within the head" or headache
enostosis (en/ost/osis) — an abnormal bony growth developed within the cavity of a bone

Lesson 9 — Reading Assignment

emplastic (em/plast/ic) — literally "pertaining to forming within"; adhesive; a constipating medicine

gangli-   swelling; knotlike mass

This root denotes relationship to a ganglion:
ganglion (gangli/on) — a normal mass of nerve cells outside of the brain and spinal column; or, an abnormal tumor or cyst consisting of tendon tissue and usually appearing on a wrist or an ankle

Examples:
ganglicocytoma (gangli/o/cyt/oma) — a tumor containing ganglion cells
ganglioplexus (gangli/o/plex/us) — a network (plexus) of nerve fibers in a ganglion
ganglionectomy (gangli/on/ectomy) — excision of a ganglion

gemin-   twin, double / paired

Examples:
gemin-   form denoting relationship to twins or pairs
geminate (gemin/ate) — paired; occurring in pairs; also called bi/gemin/al
geminus (gemin/us) — a twin
gemini (gemin/i) — twins

grad-   walk; take steps / a stage in a process

Examples:
-grade (-grad/e) — suffix indicating a series of steps; a progression
retrograde (retr/o/grad/e) — going backward
digitograde (digit/o/grad/e) — characterized by walking on the toes

gran-   grain, particle

Examples:
granul- (gran/ul-) — form denoting relationship to small particles
granule (gran/ul/e) — a small particle
granulation (gran/ul/ation) — the formation in wounds of small rounded fleshy masses
granuloma (gran/ul/oma) — a tumor composed of grainy tissue
granuloplastic (gran/ul/o/plast/ic) — forming granules

labi-   lip / any liplike structure, especially the lips of the face

The root **labi-** is the landmark reference for a lip or liplike structure; the root **cheil-** is used to designate conditions of or therapy applied to the lip.

Examples:
labium (labi/um) — a fleshy border or edge; used as a general term to designate such a structure
labial (labi/al) — pertaining to a lip; pertaining to a labium
labiodental (labi/o/dent/al) — pertaining to the lips and teeth
labiology (labi/ology) — the study of the movements of the lips in singing and speaking

later-   side / the side of the body

Examples:
lateral (later/al) — pertaining to a side; also, denoting a position farther from the middle or the midline of the body or of a structure

Lesson 9 — Reading Assignment

laterad (later/ad) — toward a side
lateroposition (later/o/position) — displacement to one side
laterality (later/al/ity) — a tendency to use the organs (hand, foot, ear, eye) of the same side

mamm-   breast

Examples:
mammi-, mammo- (mamm/i-, mamm/o-) — forms denoting relationship to the breast or the milk secreting gland in the breast of the female (the mast/aden-)
mamma (mamm/a) — name for the breast
mammary (mamm/ary) — pertaining to the breast
mamill-   an element used to denote the nipple of the breast or any nipplelike structure (note the dropping of the double "m" [mam(m)] and the use of a double "l" at the end; the literal meaning of this element is "little breast")

mamilla (mamill/a) — name for the nipple or any nipplelike structure

Comparision of **mamm-** to **mast-**:

The root **mamm-** is mostly used to designate the breast as a structure or landmark, for example:

mammose (mamm/ose) — having large breasts
mammoplasty (mamm/o/plast/y) — plastic reconstruction of the breast

The root **mast-** is used more to designate the female breast and the mammary gland (the milk-secreting gland) and the diseases and corrective procedures relating to the female breast and mammary gland.

mastalgia (mast/algia) — pain in the mammary gland
mastectomy (mast/ectomy) — excision of the breast; mammectomy

micr-   small / small size; minute, that is, "microscopic"

This root is widely used in medical terms to convey the idea of "smallness." Micr / _____ / ia or micr / _____ / y — forms used to designate abnormally small body structures, such as:

microblepharia (micr/o/blephar/ia) — small eyelids
microcephaly (micr/o/cephal/y) — small head
microcardia (micr/o/card/ia) — small heart

The root may be used to distinguish smaller from larger structures, such as:

microaden- (micr/o/aden-) — small glands, usually small lymph glands
microangi- (micr/o/angi-) — small blood vessels
microscope (micr/o/scop/e) — an instrument used to obtain a large image of small objects
microscopic (micr/o/scop/ic) — of extremely small size; visible only by the aid of a microscope
microsurgery (micr/o/surgery) — dissection of small structures under the microscope

The root can serve to illustrate some of the distinctions in the use of synonymous or related elements:

microphthalmia (micr/ophthalm/ia) — abnormal smallness of the eyes
micropsia (micr/ops/ia) — a condition in which objects are seen as smaller than they usually are
micrencephaly (micr/en/cephal/y) — abnormal smallness of the brain
micropsychia (micr/o/psych/ia) — literally "a condition of small mind"; feebleness of the mind, feeble-minded

Lesson 9 — Reading Assignment

peps-, pept-   digest / digestion

    Examples:
        pepsin (peps/in) — a substance secreted in the stomach which begins the digestive process
        peptic (pept/ic) — pertaining to digestion, such as a peptic ulcer (an ulcer is an open sore; other than a wound on the skin or some mucous membrane) which is an ulcer on the lining of the stomach; pertaining to pepsin
        -pepsia (-peps/ia) — a condition of digestion

        dyspepsia (dys/peps/ia) — faulty digestion; indigestion
        bradypepsia (brady/peps/ia) — slow digestion

peri-   about, around / surrounding; enclosing; covering

This prefix is used widely in medical terms to designate the area or space around a body part (the "vicinity" or "neighborhood"); the tissue that encloses and frequently supports or lubricates a part.

In the sense of the area or space around a part:

        periodontal (peri/odont/al) — situated or occurring around a tooth
        periosteoma (peri/oste/oma) — a morbid bony growth surrounding a bone
        periadenitis (peri/aden/itis) — inflammation of the tissues around a gland

In the sense of a tissue that covers, surrounds, or encloses a part:

        peri/o/ _____ /ium, peri/o/ _____ /eum — form used to name the enclosing or covering tissue of a part

        periosteum (peri/oste/um) — a specialized connective tissue covering all bones of the body
        pericardium (peri/card/ium) — the fibrous sac that surrounds the heart

phob-   fear / persistent abnormal fear or dread

    Examples:
        phobia (phob/ia) — name for abnormal fear
        -phobia (-phob/ia) — word termination designating abnormal fear of or aversion to the subject indicated by the preceding element to which it is affixed
        phobe, -phobe (phob/e, -phob/e) — one having a specified phobia
        phobic, -phobic (phob/ic, -phob/ic) — of the nature of or pertaining to phobia or morbid fear
        phobophobia (phob/o/phob/ia) — a condition marked by fear of one's own fear

phot-   light

    Examples:
        photic (phot/ic) — pertaining to light
        photoallergy (phot/o/allergy) — an allergic type of sensitivity to light
        photophobia (phot/o/phob/ia) — abnormal intolerance of light
        photosensitive (phot/o/sensitive) — sensitive to light
        photo-ophthalmia (phot/o/-ophthalm/ia) — blindness or severe inflammation of the eye caused by intense light such as an electric light, rays of welding arc, or reflection from snow

pleur-   pleura (membrane)
        rib, side

Lesson 9 — Reading Assignment

Examples:

pleura (pleur/a) — name for the membrane that covers the lungs and lines the thoracic (chest) cavity

pleural (pleur/al) — pertaining to the pleura

pleurisy, pleuritis, (pleur/isy, pleur/itis) — inflammation of the pleura

pleuropneumonia (pleur/o/pneumon/ia) — pleurisy complicated with pneumonia

pleurocholecystitis (pleur/o/chole/cyst/itis) — inflammation of the pleura and the gallbladder

pro- in front of; before / front part of

Examples:

prolabium (pro/labi/um) — the prominent central part of the upper lip

prolapse (pro/lapse) — a slipping forward (or out of place) of an organ or part of the body; a displacement (lapse means "a fall")

proptosis (pro/ptosis) — a forward displacement

prootic (pro/ot/ic) — situated in front of the ear

proencephalon (pro/en/cephal/on) — the front part of the brain

rachi- spinal column / spine; the backbone; the vertebral column

Examples:

rachis (rachi/s) — name for the spinal column

rachidial, rachidian (rachidi/al, rachidi/an) — pertaining to the spinal column

rachitis (rach/itis) — inflammation of the spine; a disease commonly known as rickets, in which there is a failure to form bones properly and a softening of the bones because of a lack of vitamin D

rachitic (rach/it/ic) — pertaining to or affected with rickets or rachitis

rachicentesis (rachi/centesis) — puncture into the spine

tarso- framework of the eyelid

We learned tarso- in Lesson 7 with the meaning "ankle". The element is re-introduced in order that you may remember another meaning, "framework of the eyelid".

Examples:

tarsus of the lower eyelid (tars/us) — the edge of the lower eyelid

tarsus of the upper eyelid (tars/us) — the edge of the upper eyelid

tarsitis (tars/itis) — inflammation of the tarsus or edge of the eyelid; blepharitis

Lesson 9 — Element Recognition Exercise

Separate the elements, connecting vowels, and word terminals of the following medical words by inserting a slash mark (/) between them.

Example: dorsocephalad — dors/o/cephal/ad

tarsocheiloplasty	pleuralgia
cheiropodalgia	mammectomy
calculogenesis	rachiotomy
cineplasty	topophobia
dorsalgia	photesthesis
graduated	dyscholia
granulocytopenia	cutitis
labiomycosis	encephalalgia
microangiopathy	pericerebral
peptogenic	proglossis
mammoplasia	tarsitis
lateral	cheirarthritis
rachiodynia	calcaneodynia
phagophobia	cinesalgia
photodermatosis	granulocyte
dysosteogenesis	labiology
subcutaneous	microlithiasis
encephalomeningopathy	pleurocholecystitis
mammoplasty	dysendocrinia
periglossitis	encysted
proptosis	periosteoma

Lesson 10 — Review

ELEMENT	AUDIONYM	VISUAL IMAGE	MEANING
mechano-	mechanic	See the **mechan**ic with a washing **machine** strapped on his back!	machine
dynam-	dynamite	See the **dynam**ite exploding with **power** saws bursting out of them!	power
osmo-	I smoke	See the man saying, "**I smo**ke '**O**' **do**ors."!	odor
traumat-	laundromat	See the laun**dromat** with the washers and dryers that are **wound**ed!	wound, injury
trich-	trick	See the magician performing **trick**s covered with **hair**!	hair
maxill-	makes hill	See the bulldozer that **makes hil**ls with an **upper jawbone**!	upper jawbone
an-,a-	an a	See the image of **an "A"** (the student's report card) **without** one, **not** one "A"!	without, not
phak-	vacuum cleaner	See the **vac**uum cleaner with a **lens** on it!	lens
pre-	pray	See the people of the congregation stopping to **pray in front of** the church **before** entering!	in front of, before
strict-	strict	See the **strict** parent using a rope **draw**n **tight**ly around the teenagers to control them!	to draw tight, narrowing
turbin-	turban	See the **turban shaped like a top**!	shaped like a top
ameb-	a me	See the person looking into the mirror asking "**a me**" for **change**!	change

Lesson 10 — Review

ELEMENT	AUDIONYM	VISUAL IMAGE	MEANING
semi-	semi colon	See the **semi-**colon cut in **half**!	half
neo-	kneel	See the people k**neel**ing on the **new** carpet saying, "Its **new**! It's **new**!"!	new
hormone-	harmonize	See the couple **harmon**izing with everyone heading to the **exit**!	excite or set in motion
therm-	thermometer	See the people around the **therm**ometer as it generates **heat**!	heat
syn- or sym-	cymbals	See the **cym**bals stuck **together**!	together
vuls(e)-	false	See the **false** teeth being **pull**ed by **tw**o **witch**es!	twitch or pull
post	post office	See the person who arrived at the **post** office **after** it closed!	after, behind in time
metr-	meter	See the **met**er saying, "Yo**u turn us**"!	uterus
tegument	tag you men	See the **men** playing **tag** and being **covered** with a piece of **skin**!	covering or skin
pan-	pan	See the **pan** that contains **all** the food in the house!	all
poly-	polish	See the shoe **poli**sh made of **many** colors!	many or much
ramus	ram	See the **ram** with **branch**es instead of horns!	branch
neuro-	Nero	See **Nero** being very **nervous** as Rome burns!	nerve (nervous System)

129

Lesson 10 — Worksheet

Complete the following:

ELEMENT	AUDIONYM	MEANING
mechano-	_____	_____
dynam-	_____	_____
osmo-	_____	_____
traumat-	_____	_____
trich-	_____	_____
maxill-	_____	_____
an-, a-	_____	_____
phak-	_____	_____
pre-	_____	_____
strict-	_____	_____
turbin-	_____	_____
ameb-	_____	_____
semi-	_____	_____
neo-	_____	_____
hormone-	_____	_____
therm-	_____	_____
syn- or sym-	_____	_____
vuls(e)-	_____	_____
post	_____	_____
metr-	_____	_____
tegument	_____	_____
pan-	_____	_____
poly-	_____	_____
ramus	_____	_____
neuro-	_____	_____

Lesson 10 — Reading Assignment

ameb-   change / a parasite which moves by changing shape

Examples:
  ameba, amoeba (ameb/a, amoeb/a) — a one-celled animal which moves by constantly changing its shape; amebas (amoebas) are found in soil and water and some varieties exist as parasites in human tissues and cavities
  amebic (ameb/ic) — pertaining to, or of the nature of, an ameba
  amebiasis (ameb/ia/sis) — infestation with amebas, especially with a variety that is a parasite in the intestines

an-, a-   without, not / lacking; weakness; deficiency

This is a widely used prefix which can be attached to words to indicate the negative or opposite aspect of the word to which it is prefixed. Most of the applications in medical terms carry the meaning of "without" in the sense of "lacking," "being deficient in," "weakness in."

Note: The form of the prefix is ***an-*** before vowels (a, e, i, o, u and usually h); the form is ***a-*** before all other letters (the consonants).

Examples:
  anemia (an/em/ia) — "lack of blood"; lack of red cells in the blood
  anesthesia (an/esthesia) — "lack of feeling"; unconsciousness
  avitaminosis (a/vitamin/osis) — "lack of vitamins"; a disease caused by vitamin deficiency
  atrophy (a/trophy) — "lacking development, growth"; a wasting away or a decrease in the size of a cell, tissue, organ or part due to a defect of nutrition

dynam-   power / force; strength

Examples:
  dynamic (dynam/ic) — pertaining to or exhibiting force
  adynamia (a/dynam/ia) — lack or loss of normal powers; asthenia
  myodynamic (my/o/dynam/ic) — relating to muscular force
  hyperdynamia (hyper/dynam/ia) — excessive muscle activity
  cardiodynamics (cardi/o/dynam/ics) — science of the motions and forces involved in the heart's action

hormone   to excite or set in motion / applied to a substance formed in an organ of the body (principally the glands) and carried by a body fluid to another organ or tissue where it has a specific effect such as stimulation or arousal.

Examples:
  hormonic (hormon/ic) — pertaining to or acting as a hormone; having the exciting influence of a hormone
  hormonotherapy (hormon/o/therap/y) — treatment by the use of hormones
  hyperhormonal (hyper/hormon/al) — pertaining to hormone excess
  hypohormonal (hypo/hormon/al) — pertaining to hormone deficiency

maxill-   upper jawbone

Examples:
  maxilla (maxill/a) — name of the upper jawbone. There are two such bones, the left maxilla and the right maxilla, which are joined at the center of the face.
  maxillary (maxill/ary) — pertaining to the maxilla
  maxillectomy (maxill/ectomy) — surgical removal of the maxilla
  maxillolabial (maxill/o/labi/al) — pertaining to the upper jawbone and the lip

Lesson 10 — Reading Assignment

mechano-   machine

Examples:
mechanotherapy (mechano/therap/y) — the use of mechanical apparatus (machines) in the treatment of disease; especially as an aid in performing therapeutic exercises

mechanism (mechan/ism) — this word, formed from the root mechan-, is used in medical terminology to designate a system or a mental or physical process by which some result is produced

labor mechanism (mechanism of labor) — the process involved in the expulsion of the infant and the afterbirth through the birth canal in labor

defense mechanism — any self-protective physiological reaction of an organism; in psychiatry, any behavior or thought process unconsciously brought into use by an individual to protect himself against painful or anxiety-provoking feelings and impulses

metr-   uterus / womb / hyster-; female organ for protection and nourishment of the developing young during pregnancy

Examples:
-metrium (-metr/ium) — part or layer of the uterus (womb)

myometrium (my/o/metr/ium) — the smooth muscle coat of the uterus
endometrium (end/o/metr/ium) — the mucous coat (lining) of the uterus

-metra (-metr/a) — a condition of the uterus (Note that we are accustomed to ***-ia*** as a word terminal denoting condition; the ***-a*** terminal with metr- is an exception.)

hematometra (hemat/o/metr/a) — an accumulation of blood in the uterus

Comparison of ***hyster-***, ***metr-***, ***uterus*** and ***womb***:

All of these expressions refer to the female organ containing the young during pregnancy.
womb — the common name and seldom used in medical terminology
uterus — the medical name for the structure
hyster- and ***metr-*** — used interchangeably with a tendency to use hyster- as the root to denote surgical procedures (operations) and metr- as the root denoting structural parts

neo-   new / recent

Examples:
neonatal (neo/natal) — "new born"; pertaining to the first four weeks after birth
neopathy (neo/path/y) — a new disease; a new condition or complication of disease in a patient
neoplasm (neo/plasm) — any new and abnormal growth such as a tumor

In Lesson 1 we learned plast- and in Lesson 6, -plasia. Both of these elements contain the root plas- which denotes the idea of forming or formation. The suffix -plas/m indicates formative or formed material. In medical terms the reference is usually to the formation of cells or tissues.

neuro-   nerve or nervous system

Examples:
neuron (neur/on) — a nerve cell
neural (neur/al) — pertaining to a nerve or the nerves
psychoneurosis, neurosis (psych/o/neur/osis, neur/osis) — both terms are used to designate any

Lesson 10 — Reading Assignment

of various psychic or mental disturbances, characterized by one or several of such reactions as: anxiety, compulsions and obsessions, phobias, depression, etc.

-neuria (-neur/ia) — suffix denoting a condition of nerve function

dysneuria (dys/neur/ia) — impairment of the nerve function
gastrohyperneuria (gastr/o/hyper/neur/ia) — excessive activity of the nerves of the stomach

-neurium (-neur/ium) — suffix denoting a nerve tissue

perineurium (peri/neur/ium) — the connective tissue cover around the nerve fibers

osmo-   odor / smell; the sense of smell

Examples:
osmics (osm/ics) — the science that deals with the sense of smell; the study of odors
osmatic, -osmatic (osmat/ic, -osmat/ic) — pertaining to the sense of smell
anosmatic (an/osmat/ic) — having no sense of or only an imperfect sense of smell
-osmia (-osm/ia) — a condition of the sense of smell

anosmia (an/osm/ia) — absence of the sense of smell
hyposmia (hyp/osm/ia) — abnormally decreased sensitiveness to odor

pan-   all / completely; the whole of (also pant-)

Examples:
panhysterectomy (pan/hyster/ectomy) — the removal by surgery of the whole of the uterus
pancarditis (pan/card/itis) — inflammation of all of the heart, that is, the outer covering (peri/card/itis), the muscular wall (my/o/card/itis) and the lining of the cavities of the heart (end/o/card/itis)
pantosomatous (pant/o/somat/ous) — pertaining or relating to the whole body
pantalgia (pant/algia) — pain over the whole body

phak-   lens / the crystalline lens of the eye, that is, the transparent body of tissue behind the pupil of the eye which focuses the incoming light rays

Examples:
phakitis, also phacitis (phak/itis, phac/itis) — inflammation of the crystalline lens of the eye
phacocele (phac/o/cele) — the displacement of the eye lens from its proper place; hernia of the eye lens
phacocyst- (phac/o/cyst-) — form denoting relationship to the sac enclosing the crystalline lens of the eye

poly-   many or much / sometimes with the idea of excessive

Examples:
polyacoustic (poly/acoust/ic) — "much sound"; increasing or intensifying sound
polycythemia (poly/cyt/hem/ia) — excessive number of red corpuscles in the blood
polyemia (poly/em/ia) — excessive amount of blood in the body

The prefix may be used to indicate a condition involving many of a kind of body part or organ:
polyadenitis (poly/aden/itis) — inflammation of several or many glands; similarly poly/aden/oma, poly/aden/o/path/y, poly/aden/osis
polydysplasia (poly/dys/plas/ia) — faulty development in several types of tissue or several organs or systems of organs

Lesson 10 — Reading Assignment

post   after, behind in time / also, situated behind (behind in place)

   Examples:
   postpneumonia (post/pneumon/ia) — following pneumonia
   postoral (post/or/al) — situated behind the mouth
   postnatal (post/natal) — after the occurrence of birth
   poster-   form denoting relationship to the rear part or back part

       posterior (poster/ior) — situated in the back part of, or affecting the back part of an organ
       posteriad (poster/i/ad) — toward the posterior part of the body
       posterolateral (poster/o/later/al) — situated behind and to one side

pre-   in front of; before / situated before, or in front of; occurring before, or prior to, or earlier than

   Examples:
   prerenal (pre/ren/al) — situated in front of the kidney
   prepartal (pre/part/al) — occurring before, or just previous, to labor
   prenatal (pre/nat/al) — existing or occurring before birth
   preoperative (pre/operative) — preceding an operation
   precranial (pre/crani/al) — in the front part of the cranium

ramus   branch / a branch or branchlike projecting part

There are many networks in the body which can be described as branching, for example, the nervous system, the circulatory system (arteries, veins and capillaries). These may be called branches or, with the addition of complex Latin terms, be called ramus. In lesson 6 we learned dendr- meaning "branch." Dendr- is used almost exclusively to indicate the branch of a nerve cell. All other branches are designated as ramus.

   Examples:
   ramitis (ram/itis) — inflammation of root
   ramose (ram/ose) — branching; having many branches

semi-   half / one-half; partially

   Examples:
   semilunar (semi/lunar) — resembling a crescent or halfmoon
   semimalignant (semi/malign/ant) — somewhat (partially) malignant
   seminormal (semi/normal) — one-half the normal

strict-   to draw tight; narrowing

   Examples:
   stricture (strict/ure) — the abnormal narrowing of a canal, duct or passage

       spastic stricture (spast/ic strict/ure) — a stricture due to a muscle spasm

   stricturotomy (strict/ur/otomy) — the cutting of a stricture

syn- or sym-   together

   Examples:
   syndesis (syn/desis) — a "binding together"; the fusion of a joint; arthrodesis
   syndactyly (syn/dactyl/y) — "finger (digit) togetherness"; the most common congenital defect, affecting the hand in which adjacent digits are more or less attached to each other by a membranous web

Lesson 10 — Reading Assignment

symphysis (sym/phy/sis) — a "natural togetherness"; a type of joint in which the connected bones are firmly united such as the joint formed by the various bone parts in the hip

synalgia (syn/algia) — "pain together"; pain experienced in one place as the result of a soreness or injury in another place

tegument   skin or covering

The word tegument is a shortened form for integument which generally means "a covering" but is widely used to denote the skin.

Examples:
integumentary (integument/ary) — pertaining to or composed of skin; serving as a covering, like the skin

the integumentary system (sometimes called common integument) — a term used to designate the entire covering of the body including, not only the skin, but the other body coverings: hair, nails and the skin glands, including the breast, or mammary gland

therm-   heat

Examples:
thermal, thermic (therm/al, therm/ic) — pertaining to or characterized by heat

-thermia, -thermy (-therm/ia, -therm/y) — a state of heat; the generation of heat

diathermy (dia/therm/y) — the generation of heat in the body tissues for medical or surgical purposes, usually by the application of electrical currents (**dia-** is a prefix meaning "through" so that, literally, diathermy means "the act of heating through")

hyperthermia (hyper/therm/ia) — an abnormally high body temperature; fever

traumat-   wound; injury / shock; stress

This element is used in the form traumat- to denote relationship to a wound or injury (a trauma).

Examples:
trauma (traum/a) — (1) a bodily injury or wound caused by the application of external force or violence (injuries such as sprains, bruises, fractures, dislocations, concussions, burns, etc.) (2) a psychological or emotional stress or blow that may produce disordered feelings or behavior

psychic trauma (psych/ic traum/a) — an emotional shock that makes a lasting impression on the mind, especially the subconscious mind

traumatic (traumat/ic) — pertaining to, occurring as the result of, or causing trauma

trich-   hair

Examples:
-trichia, -trichosis (-trich/ia, -trich/osis) — condition of the hair

leukotrichia (leuk/o/trich/ia) — whiteness of the hair
sclerotrichia (scler/o/trich/ia) — hard, dry state of the hair
atrichosis (a/trich/osis) — absence of the hair; baldness

trichoesthesia (trich/o/esthesia) — "hair feeling"; the sense by which one perceives that the hair of the skin is being touched

trichogenous (trich/o/gen/ous) — promoting the growth of hair

Lesson 10 — Reading Assignment

turbin-   shaped like a top / spiral-shaped

Used principally in medical terms with reference to a turbinate which is one of several spiral spongy bony projections in the nasal passages (the nostrils).

Examples:
   turbinal (turbin/al) — shaped like a top; one of the turbinates
   turbinotomy (turbin/otomy) — the surgical cutting of a turbinate
   turbinectomy (turbin/ectomy) — the surgical removal of a turbinate bone

-vuls(e)   twitch or pull / pluck; tear loose

This element, the root of which is vuls-, is most familiar in convulse and convulsion applied to the violent, irregular motion of a limb or other part of the body due to involuntary contraction of the muscle (the prefix **con-** means "together"; the literal translation of convuls- is "a pulling together").

The root also appears in avulsion (sometimes evulsion) which describes the forcible tearing or pulling out of a part in surgery (the prefix **a-** is a form of **ab-** meaning "from" or "away from" which will be discussed more fully in Lesson 11; the literal translation of avuls- is "pulling away from").
   nerve avulsion (a/vuls/ion) — the operation of pulling a nerve from its origin
   avulsion, nail plate (a/vuls/ion) — the pulling out of a diseased or infected outer layer of the nail of a finger or toe

Lesson 10 — Element Recognition Exercise

Separate the elements, connecting vowels, and word terminals of the following medical words by inserting a slash mark (/) between them.

Example: trichorrhexis — trich/o/rrhexis

dynamogenesis

osmesthesia

traumatopathy

trichotrophy

maxillectomy

anesthesia

phacosclerosis

pretympanic

stricturotomy

turbinectomy

ameboid

neophrenia

hormonogenesis

thermohyperesthesia

syndactylism

postcardiotomy

metrophlebitis

panhematopenia

polytrichia

neurotrophasthenia

turbinotomy

ameba

neophobia

thermalgesia

synchilia

metrocolpocele

pancytolysis

polypathia

neurootology

dynamoscopy

osmophobia

traumatologist

trichorrhexis

maxillitis

analgesia

phacomalacia

precostal

thermolysis

synosteology

metrostenosis

polycheiria

neurotrauma

Lesson 11 — Review

ELEMENT	AUDIONYM	VISUAL IMAGE	MEANING
thromb-	trombone	See the **tromb**one with a **lump** or a **clot** stuck in it!	lump, clot
ab-	Abe	See **Abe** sneaking **away from** the Capitol to tie k**not**s!	away from, not
-plegia	pledge	See the people **pledg**ing allegiance to the flag and becoming **paralyzed**!	paralysis
ante-	ant tea	See the **ant** drinking **tea** with the **beef** and **oar** in it!	before
thel-	the "L"	See **the "L"** with a **nipple** stuck on it!	nipple
ex-	eggs	See the **eggs** jumping **out** of the carton and running **away**!	out, away from
lien-	line (clothes)	See the clothes**line** with students on it having a **spelli**ng bee!	spleen
tumor	two more	See Ma holding **two more** children as the bed is **swelling**!	swelling
vestibule	vest bull	See the **vest** on the **bull**. It is an **entrance**!	entrance
puer-	pure (gold)	See the **pure** gold **child**!	child
sarc-	shark	See the **shark** made of **flesh**!	flesh
proli-	parolee	See the **parole**e jumping **off** the **spring**!	offspring
macro-	macaroni	See the **macaro**ni that is very very **large**!	large

138

Lesson 11 — Review

ELEMENT	AUDIONYM	VISUAL IMAGE	MEANING
lal-	lolly (pop)	See the **lol**lypop giving a **speech**!	speech
intra-	introduce	See the person being **intro**duced to someone **within** the man!	within
inter-	interpreter	See the **inter**preter. She is a **bee** in **tweed**!	between
infra-	infra red oven	See the **infra** red oven with a **bee** on its **knee**s!	beneath
cryo-	cry	See the baby **cry**ing because it is **cold**. It is on an igloo!	cold
mal-	mall	See the **mal**l with baseball **bat**s shopping!	bad
glom-	glow	See the **glo**w in the sky with **ball**s falling out of it!	ball
tens-	tents	See the **tents stretch**ed!	stretch
spas-	space	See the **space** vehicle **pulling** another vehicle with someone **drawing** in it!	pull, draw
somni-	"saw my knee"	See the woman saying, "He **saw my knee**" because I was **sleep**ing!	sleep
pharmac-	farm axe	See the farmer with the **"farm axe"** made of a **drug**store!	drug
lumbo-	lumber	See the **lumb**er with the **lions** coming out of it!	loins

Lesson 11 — Worksheet

Complete the following:

ELEMENT	AUDIONYM	MEANING
thromb-		
ab-		
-plegia		
ante-		
thel-		
ex-		
lien-		
tumor		
vestibule		
puer-		
sarc-		
proli-		
macro-		
lal-		
intra-		
inter-		
infra-		
cryo-		
mal-		
glom-		
tens-		
spas-		
somni-		
pharmac-		
lumbo-		

Lesson 11 — Reading Assignment

ab- away from

This prefix takes the form **a-** before m, p and v and **abs-** before c and t.

Examples:
abnormal (ab/normal) — away from normal; departing from normal
abneural (ab/neur/al) — passing from a nerve (usually to a muscle)
avulsion (a/vuls/ion) — "a pulling away from"; This word was discussed in Lesson 10 under -vulse but is introduced here to help in understanding the "away from" meaning of **a-** as a form of **ab-**.

ante- before / before in time (occurring before); before in space (situated in front of or at the front of)

Examples:
antepartum (ante/part/um) — occurring before birth
antelocation (ante/location) — the forward (toward the front) displacement of an organ

This prefix appears in a frequently used form **anter/o-** which is restricted to the meaning "before in space (situated in front)" or "forward" and usually carrying the idea of direction.

anterior (anter/ior) — situated more toward the forward part of an organ; used freely to designate the belly surface of the body
anteroposterior (anter/o/poster/ior) — from front to back

cryo- cold

Examples:
cryotherapy (cryo/therap/y) — the therapeutic use of cold
hematocryal (hemat/o/cry/al) — cold blooded
cryosurgery (cryo/surgery) — the destruction of tissue by extreme cold as, for example, the treatment of malignant tumors of the skin
cryoextraction (cryo/extraction) — the application of low temperature in the removal of a body part such as a cataract

ex- out; away from / out of; outside of

the element **ex-** may appear in several forms:

exo- meaning "outside"; "outward"; "outer"

exogenic (exo/gen/ic) — "produced outside"; developed or originating outside the body
exopathy (exo/path/y) — "disease outside"; a disease originating in some cause lying outside the body

extra- meaning "outside of"; "beyond"

extracardial (extra/cardi/al) — outside the heart
extrahepatic (extra/hepat/ic) — situated or occurring outside the liver

ecto- situated on the outside; outside

ectosteal (ect/oste/al) — pertaining to or situated on the outside of a bone
ectocytic (ecto/cyt/ic) — outside the cell

141

Lesson 11 — Reading Assignment

Examples:

exostosis (ex/ost/osis) — a condition (bony growth) projecting outward from the surface of a bone

extensor (ex/tens/or) — that which stretches (extends) as, for example, a muscle which extends a joint

glom-   ball / a rounded mass; a cluster; in the form of a ball; a tuft

This root is used chiefly in medical terminology to denote two kinds of small anatomical structures:

glomus (glom/us) — a small round anatomical (normal) swelling made up of tiny blood vessels

glomic (glom/ic) — pertaining to a glomus

glomerulus (glomer/ul/us) — a tufted structure or a cluster generally composed of blood vessels or nerve fibers; used principally to designate coils of blood vessels in the kidney

glomerul- (glomer/ul-) — form for a glomerulus
glomerular (glomer/ul/ar) — pertaining to or of the nature of a glomerulus

infra-   beneath / situated or occurring below or beneath

Examples:

inframammary (infra/mamm/ary) — situated below the mammary gland
inframaxillary (infra/maxill/ary) — beneath the jaw
infracostal (infra/cost/al) — beneath the ribs or beneath a rib
infrapsychic (infra/psych/ic) — below the psychic (mind) level; non-thinking; automatic

inter-   between / situated, formed or occurring between

This prefix is used widely to designate a location between or among the parts or structures named in the second element to which it is affixed.

Examples:

interlabial (inter/labi/al) — between lips
interosseous (inter/oss/eous) — between bones
intermuscular (inter/muscul/ar) — between muscles
interdigital (inter/digit/al) — between adjacent fingers or toes

intra-   within / situated within

This prefix is used widely with the meanings "situated within" or "occurring within."

Examples:

intraspinal (intra/spin/al) — situated or occurring within the vertebral column
intraoperative (intra/operative) — performed or occurring within the course of a surgical operation

A variation of intra- is the prefix **intro-** carrying the meaning "into"; frequently "insertion into."

lal-   speech / babbling

Examples:

lalopathy (lal/o/path/y) — any disorder of speech
lalophobia (lal/o/phob/ia) — fear or extreme dislike of speaking (stage fright), often associated with stuttering

Lesson 11 — Reading Assignment

-lalia (-lal/ia) — a speech disorder

echolalia (echo/lal/ia) — the meaningless repitition by a patient of words addressed to him

rhinolalia (rhin/o/lal/ia) — a nasal quality of voice due to some disorder or defect of the nasal passages

bradylalia (brady/lal/ia) — abnormally slow speech due to a brain disorder

lien-   spleen / the fist-sized organ near the stomach in the upper part of the abdomen which modifies and stores blood

Examples:

lienal (lien/al) — pertaining to the spleen

lien — name for the spleen

gastrolienal (gastr/o/lien/al) — pertaining to the stomach and the spleen

lienorenal (lien/o/ren/al) — pertaining to the spleen and the kidney

lumbo-   loins / the sides of the back lying on each side of the spinal column between the end of the ribs and the hipbone

Examples:

lumbar (lumb/ar) — pertaining to the loins

lumbago, lumbodynia (lumb/ago, lumb/odyn/ia) — pain in the lumbar region; "lower back pains"

dorsolumbar (dors/o/lumb/ar) — pertaining to the back and loins

supralumbar (supra/lumb/ar) — situated above the loins

sublumbar (sub/lumb/ar) — situated below the loins

macro-   large / enlargement

This root carries the meaning large or of abnormal size or length. The form for abnormal size or length is usually macr/ _____ /ia or macr/ _____ /y.

Examples:

macropsia (macr/ops/ia) — "large vision"; a disturbance of vision in which objects are seen as larger than they really are

macrophthalmia (macr/ophthalm/ia) — "large eyes"; abnormal enlargement of the eyeballs

macrostomia (macro/stom/ia) — "big mouth"; greatly exaggerated width of the mouth

macrotooth (macro/tooth) — an abnormally large tooth

macrodontia (macr/odont/ia) — abnormal increase in the size of the teeth

mal-   bad / irregular; abnormal; faulty; poor (in the sense of inadequate or insufficient)

Examples:

maldigestion (mal/digestion) — faulty or impaired digestion

malformation (mal/formation) — defective or abnormal formation; deformity

malpractice (mal/practice) — improper or injurious practice; unskillful and faulty medical or surgical treatment

pharmac-   drug / medicinal drug; medicine

Examples:

pharmacy (pharmac/y) — the art of preparing, compounding and dispensing medicines; a drug store (in the sense of a store or shop in which prescription drugs are prepared and dispensed)

pharmacal (pharmac/al) — pertaining to pharmacy

pharmacopsychosis (pharmac/o/psych/osis) — a term for any one of the group of mental diseases due to alcohol, drugs or poison

photopharmacology (phot/o/pharmac/ology) — the study of the effects of light and other radiations on drugs

Lesson 11 — Reading Assignment

-plegia   paralysis / a stroke; a loss of power

Examples:
   panplegia (pan/plegia) — (also pam/plegia) total paralysis
   hemiplegia (hemi/plegia) — paralysis of one side of the body

proli-   offspring / production

Examples:
   prolific (proli/fic) — fruitful; productive (**-fic** is an ending meaning "causing." "bringing about")
   proliferous (proli/fer/ous) — characterized by the production of offspring (**-ferous** is an ending meaning "bearing," "producing")

puer-   child / children

Examples:
   puerile (puer/ile) — pertaining to childhood or to children; childish
   puerper- (puer/per-) — combination denoting relationship to childbirth

      puerpera (puer/per/a) — a woman who has just given birth to a child; a new mother
      puerperium (puer/per/ium) — the period or state of confinement after labor

sarc-   flesh / fleshy material

   sarcolysis (sarc/o/lysis) — disintegration of the soft tissues; disintegration of flesh
   sarcocele (sarc/o/cete) — any fleshy swelling
   sarcoma, -sarcoma (sarc/oma, -sarc/oma) — a tumor made up of fleshy substance
   adenochondrosarcoma (aden/o/chondr/o/sarc/oma) — a tumor containing the elements of adenoma, chondroma and sarcoma, that is a tumor blended of glandular, cartilaginous and fleshy substances

somni-   sleep

Examples:
   somnipathy (somni/path/y) — any disorder of sleep; a hypnotic trance
   somniferous (somni/fer/ous) — inducing or causing sleep (**-ferous** is an ending meaning "producing")
   insomnia (in/somn/ia) — inability to sleep; also called hyposomnia
   hypersomnia (hyper/somn/ia) — "excessive sleep"; uncontrollable drowsiness; abnormally excessive sleep
   somnolence (somnol/ence) — sleepiness

spas-   pull; draw / contraction

A form of this root **-spasm**, was learned in Lesson 1 with the meaning "involuntary contraction." The root **spas-** indicates any of the involuntary muscular movements ranging in severity from mild but annoying muscle twitches through cramps to convulsion. The most frequent forms in which the root appears in addition to spasm are:
   -spasia (-spas/ia) — a condition of muscular contraction

      myospasia (my/o/spas/ia) — a spasmodic condition in which rigidity of the muscles is followed immediately by relaxation

   -spasmia (-spasm/ia) — a disease characterized by spasms

Lesson 11 — Reading Assignment

myospasmia (my/o/spasm/ia) — disease characterized by uncontrollable muscle spasms

spastic (spast/ic) — of the nature of or characterized by spasms

tens- stretch

The key to this element lies in the root **ten-** which carries a basic meaning of "stretch" and is applied in medical terminology to convey the idea of "stretcher" (a thing that stretches) or "stretching" (the act, or action, of extending or reaching out.) The root appears in several forms:

tendon (tend/on) — any of the cords of tough, fibrous connective tissue which muscle fibers end and by which muscles are attached to bones or other parts

teno-, tenono-, tenonto- (ten/o, tenon/o-, tenont/o) — forms denoting relationship to tendons
tenotomy (ten/otomy) — the cutting of a tendon
tenonitis or tenontitis (tenon/itis, tenont/itis) — inflammation of a tendon

tensor (tens/or) — any muscle that stretches, or tenses, some part of the body

tension (tens/ion) — the act or condition of being stretched or strained

muscular tension (tens/ion) — the condition of moderate tension produced by stretching a muscle
neurotension (neur/o/tens/ion) — the surgical stretching of a nerve

thel- nipple / a thin layer of tissue

Primarily the root denotes a nipple or teat.

Examples:
thelium (thel/ium) — name for the nipple
thelitis (thel/itis) — inflammation of the nipple

The meaning of the root has been extended in the suffix combination **-thelium** which denotes a tissue forming a covering or lining of a body surface.

epithelium (epi/thel/ium) — a tissue covering surfaces, forming glands, and lining most cavities of the body
endothelium (end/o/thel/ium) — the layer of cells (tissue) lining the inside of blood and lymph vessels, of the heart, and some other closed cavities

thromb- lump; clot / a thickening; coagulation

This root is principally applied to the clotting properties and problems of the blood.

Examples:
thrombus (thromb/us) — a clot in a blood vessel or one of the cavities of the heart, formed by coagulation of the blood
thrombin (thromb/in) — a substance in the blood which helps the blood to clot (such as in a wound)
thrombosis (thromb/osis) — the formation of a blood clot in a blood vessel or organ
thrombocyte (thromb/o/cyt/e) — "a clotting cell"; a small cell in the body which plays an important part in clotting

Lesson 11 — Reading Assignment

tumor   swelling; a circumscribed, usually non-inflammatory, swelling or mass of new tissue growth arising from existing tissue but developing independently of that tissue's normal rate and structure.

You have learned that **tumor** is the meaning of the elements **-oma,** taught in Lesson 1, and **onco-,** taught in Lesson 5. The use of the word has been covered in the Reading Assignments for both. Tumor is included in this lesson to provide you the way of remembering that it means swelling.

vestibule   entrance; a space or cavity around or forming the entrance to a canal or other space

Examples:
vestibular (vestibul/ar) — pertaining to a vestibule
vestibule of the mouth — that portion of the oral cavity (cavity of the mouth) between the inside of the lips and cheeks and the outside of the teeth and gums
buccal vestibule — that portion of the vestibule of the mouth which lies between the inside of the <u>cheeks</u> and the outside of the teeth and gums
labial vestibule — that portion of the vestibule of the mouth which lies between the inside of the <u>lips</u> and the outside of the teeth and gums
vestibular labyrinth — pertaining to one of two chambers of the inner ear known as the labyrinth

Lesson 11 — Element Recognition Exercise

Separate the elements, connecting vowels, and word terminals of the following medical words by inserting a slash mark (/) between them.

Example: vestibuloplasty — vestibul/o/plast/y

thrombocyst	sarcomyces
ablactation	macroesthesia
phrenoplegia	laloplegia
theleplasty	intraosseous
exenteritis	interchondral
tumorigenesis	infrapsychic
vestibulotomy	cryalgesia
sarcadenoma	glomoid
prolific	somnific
macronychia	pharmacomania
laloneurosis	lumbodynia
intraleukocyte	thrombogenesis
interpalpebral	ablepharia
infracostal	paraplegia
cryesthesia	thelalgia
malpractice	exodontia
glomangioma	lienocele
hypertension	inframaxillary
somnipathy	lumbodorsal
pharmacodynamics	lienorenal
lumbocostal	lalophobia

Lesson 12— Review

ELEMENT	MEANING
arter-	artery
appendic-	appendix
thyro-	thyroid
splen-	spleen
ovario-	ovary
adreno-	adrenal gland
basi-	base
pelvis	pelvis
vena-	vein
urethra	urethra
utero-	uterus
sacro-	sacrum
pharyng-	pharynx

Lesson 12— Review

ELEMENT	MEANING
duodeno-	duodenum
ureter	ureter
laryng-	larynx
bronch-	bronchus
col-	colon
esophag-	esophagus
bi-	two, double, both
tri-	three
ile-	ileum
ili-	ilium
lig-	ligament
therap-	therapy

Lesson 12 — Worksheet

Complete the following:

ELEMENT	MEANING
arter-	_____
appendic-	_____
thyro-	_____
splen-	_____
ovario-	_____
adreno-	_____
basi-	_____
pelvis	_____
vena-	_____
urethra	_____
utero-	_____
sacro-	_____
pharyng-	_____
duodeno-	_____
ureter	_____
laryng-	_____
bronch-	_____
col-	_____
esophag-	_____
bi-	_____
tri-	_____
ile-	_____
ili-	_____
lig-	_____
therap-	_____

Lesson 12 — Reading Assignment

adreno-   adrenal gland

The "near or toward the kidney" glands; either of a pair of endocrine ("secreting within") glands lying immediately above the kidney, producing a variety of hormones.

Examples:
   adrenal (adren/al) — situated near the kidney; an adrenal gland
   adrenogenous (adren/o/gen/ous) — produced or arising in the adrenals
   adrenalopathy (adren/al/o/path/y) — any disease of the adrenal glands; also called adrenopathy

appendic-   appendix

An outgrowth of an organ, especially a small, saclike appendage extending from the large intestine which is commonly called "the appendix" but is technically termed the vermiform appendix (the element **vermi-** means "worm," therefore, because of its shape, "the worm-shaped appendix"). See scol- in Reading Assignment of Lesson 14.
A patient may have appendic/e/algia (or append/algia) accompanied by appendic/itis which is relieved by the performance of an append/ectomy.

Example:
   appendiceal (appendic/e/al) — pertaining to an appendix; also appendic/ul/ar

arter-   artery

Any one of the system of large, thick-walled tubes which carry blood directly from the heart to the principal parts of the body (as opposed to a vein which carries blood back to the heart).

Examples:
   arterial (arter/ial) — pertaining to an artery or the arteries
   arteriectasis (arteri/ectasis) — dilatation of an artery
   arteriectopy (arteri/ec/top/y) — displacement of an artery from its normal location
   arteriosclerosis (arteri/o/scler/osis) — hardening (sclerosis) and thickening of the arteries

basi-   base

The thing or part on which something rests; lowest part or bottom; foundation.

Examples:
   basal (bas/al) — pertaining to or situated near a base; fundamental
   basilysis (basi/lysis) — the crushing of the base of the fetal skull to facilitate delivery
   basiotripsy (basi/o/tripsy) — the crushing of the fetal head to facilitate delivery
   basis (bas/is) — the lower, basic, or fundamental of an object; used as a general term to designate the base of a structure, organ, or part opposite to, or distinguished from, the apex (apic-) or tip

bi-   two, double, both

Also twice, doubly, in pairs

Examples:
   bigeminy (bi/gemin/y) — the condition of occurring in pairs such as the occurrence of two beats of the pulse in rapid succession
   bipedal (bi/ped/al) — with, or pertaining to, both feet
   birhinia (bi/rhin/ia) — double nose
   biramus (bi/ramus) — consisting of or possessing two branches

Lesson 12 — Reading Assignment

This prefix may also appear in the form *bin-* meaning "two" or "both."

    binaural (bin/aur/al) — pertaining to both ears; also bin/ot/ic
    binocular (bin/ocul/ar) — pertaining to both eyes

bronch-   bronchus

Either of the two main branches from the trachea or windpipe which carry air into the lungs. The plural of bronchus (that is, the left bronchus and right bronchus taken together) is bronchi. The point at which the bronchi branch from the trachea is named the tracheal bifurcation (furca, Lesson 8).

Examples:
    bronchial (bronch/i/al) — pertaining to the bronchi
    bronchitis (bronch/itis) — inflammation of the bronchial tubes
    bronchopneumonia (bronch/o/pneumon/ia) — a name given to an inflammation of the lungs, which usually begins in the end of the bronchi
    bronchopleuropneumonia (bronch/o/pleur/o/pneumon/ia) — pneumonia complicated by bronchitis and pleurisy

col-   colon

The largest section of the large intestine.

Examples:
    colic (col/ic) — pertaining to the colon; also used to denote acute abdominal pain
    colocentesis (col/o/centesis) — surgical perforation (puncture) of the colon; also called col/i/puncture and col/o/puncture
    colopexy (col/o/pexy) — fixation of a bend of the colon to the abdominal wall
    colopexotomy (col/o/pex/otomy) — fixation and incision of the colon

duodeno-   duodenum

The first section of the small intestine immediately following the stomach.

Examples:
    duodenal (duoden/al) — of, pertaining to, or situated in the duodenum
    duodenocholangeitis (duoden/o/chol/ange/itis) — inflammation of the duodenum and common bile duct
    duodenocholecystostomy (duoden/o/chole/cyst/ostomy) — surgical creation of an opening (communication) between the gallbladder and the duodenum

esophag-   esophagus

The tube through which food passes from the pharynx to the stomach; the gullet.

Note: exophag- is a combination of two elements, the prefix *eso-* meaning "inner, inward" and *phage* (Lesson 8) meaning "to eat" (swallowing); just as the mouth and throat provide the "outer swallowing" of food destined for digestion in the stomach, the esophagus takes care of the "inner swallowing," the final stage of passing food to the stomach.

Examples:
    esophageal (esophag/e/al) — pertaining to or belonging to the esophagus
    esophagoptosis (esophag/o/ptosis) — prolapse (falling down or downward displacement of the esophagus)
    esophagocele (esophag/o/cele) — abnormal distention of the esophagus; hernia of the eso-

phagus; protrusion of the mucous and submucous coats of the esophagus through a rupture in the muscular coat, producing a pouch or sac

esophagomyotomy (esophag/o/my/otomy) — incision through the muscular coat of the esophagus

ile-   ileum

The lowest part of the small intestine, opening into the large intestine.

ileal (ile/al) — pertaining to the ileum

ileocystoplasty (ile/o/cyst/o/plast/y) — suture of a segment of the ileum to the urinary bladder to increase the bladder size and capacity

ileoileostomy (ile/o/ile/ostomy) — surgical creation of an opening between two parts of the ileum

ili-   ilium

The flat, uppermost portion of the three sections of the hipbone.

Examples:

iliac (ili/ac) — pertaining to the ilium

iliocostal (ili/o/cost/al) — pertaining to the ilium and the ribs

iliolumbocosto-abdominal (ili/o/lumb/o/cost/o-abdomin/al) — pertaining to the iliac, lumbar, costal and abdominal regions

laryng-   larynx

The structure of muscle and cartilage just below the pharynx. It helps to form what is commonly termed the "adam's apple." It acts in three ways: (1) as a passageway for air to the lungs; (2) as an aid in swallowing; (3) as the "voice box," that is the container of the vocal cords which aid in the formation of sounds.

Examples:

laryngeal (laryng/e/al) — of or pertaining to the larynx

laryngology (laryng/ology) — that branch of medicine which has to do with the throat. Note: Although, technically, the larynx is only part of the throat, laryngology embraces all parts of the throat. The throat can be described as that part of the neck in front of the spinal column, including the passage through it. It contains the pharynx, the larynx, the trachea and the upper part of the esophagus.

otolaryngology (ot/o/laryng/ology) — otology (the study of the ear) and laryngology (the study of the throat) considered as a single specialty

rhinolaryngology (rhin/o/laryng/ology) — rhinology (the study of the nose) and laryngology considered as a single specialty

otorhinolaryngology (ot/o/rhin/o/laryng/ology) — otology, rhinology and laryngology considered as a single specialty; also designated by the abbreviation E.N.T.

lig-   ligament

The element lig- carries the meanings "tie" or "bind." A lig/ament is a band of tough tissue connecting (tying) bones or holding (binding) organs in place.

Examples:

ligate (lig/ate) — to bind or tie with a ligature

ligature (lig/at/ure) — a thread or wire for surgical tying

ligation (lig/at/ion) — the application of a ligature

Lesson 12 — Reading Assignment

ovario-   ovary

Ovary was discussed in Lesson 5 and described as the "egg case"; either of the pair of female reproductive glands producing eggs and sex hormones.

Examples:
    ovarian (ovar/ian) — pertaining to an ovary or the ovaries
    ovarin (ovar/in) — an ovarian hormone
    ovariocentesis (ovari/o/centesis) — puncture of the ovary
    ovarioncus (ovari/onc/us) — a tumor of the ovary
    ovariorrhexis (ovari/o/rrhexis) — rupture of an ovary

pelvis   pelvis

Any basinlike or funnel-shaped structure, specifically the basinlike cavity formed by the ring of bones in the hip or pelvic girdle; it is formed by the hipbone together with the sacrum (the bone before the tailbone), supporting the spinal column and resting upon the legs.

Examples:
    pelvic (pelv/ic) — pertaining to the pelvis
    pelvitherm (pelv/i/therm) — an apparatus for applying heat to the pelvic organs through the vagina
    pelvospondylitis (pelv/o/spondyl/itis) — inflammation of the pelvic portion of the spine
    pelviotomy (pelvi/otomy) — the operation of cutting the pelvis at any point to facilitate delivery

pharyng-   pharynx

The pharynx is the muscular and membranous cavity of the digestive tube (digestive system), leading from the mouth and nasal passages to the larynx and esophagus. It is about five inches long and serves as a passage for air from the nose and mouth; it also is the passage through which food is swallowed after leaving the mouth.

Examples:
    pharyngeal (pharyng/e/al) — pertaining to the pharynx
    pharyngocele (pharyng/o/cele) — hernial protrusion of a part of the pharynx; also called pharyng/o/ectasis
    pharyngalgia (pharyng/algia) — pain in the pharynx, also called pharyng/odyn/ia
    pharyngomycosis (pharyng/o/myc/osis) — any fungus disease of the pharynx
    pharyngosalpingitis (pharyng/o/salping/itis) — inflammation of the pharynx and the eustachian tube

sacro-   sacrum

A thick, triangular bone of the vertebral column; the bone above the "tailbone"; it joins with the hip bones to form the back part of the pelvis.

Examples:
    sacral (sacr/al) — pertaining to the sacrum; the region around the sacrum
    sacrad (sacr/ad) — toward the sacrum or sacral region
    sacroplex (sacr/o/plex) — the plexus (network of nerves) stemming from the sacrum

splen-   spleen

The spleen has already been discussed in Lesson 11 under lien-.

Lesson 12 — Reading Assignment

Examples:
   splenohepatomegaly (splen/o/hepat/o/megal/y) — enlargement of the spleen and the liver
   splenogenous (splen/o/gen/ous) — produced in or formed by the spleen
   splenokeratosis (splen/o/kerat/osis) — hardening of the spleen
   splenolysis (splen/o/lysis) — destruction of spleen tissue
   laparosplenotomy (lapar/o/splen/otomy) — the operation of making an incision into the side to gain access to the spleen, usually for the purpose of draining a cyst or abscess of the spleen

therap-   therapy

The treatment of disease or of any physical or mental disorder by medical or physical means, usually excluding surgery.

Examples:
   therapeutics (therap/eutics) — the science and art of healing
   therapist (therap/ist) — a person skilled in the treatment of disease

thyro-   thyroid

Thyroid may be used to indicate a part such as a cartilage, artery, nerve, etc., in the region of the thyroid gland. The thyroid gland (thyr/o/aden-) is a large endocrine gland lying in front of and on either side of the windpipe (the trachea). It secretes a hormone which regulates body growth and metabolism.

Examples:
   hypothyroidism (hypo/thyroid/ism) — deficiency of thyroid activity or the condition resulting therefrom; also called hypo/thyroid/osis
   hyperthyroidism (hyper/thyroid/ism) — hyperactivity (excess activity) of the thyroid gland; also called hyper/thyroid/osis
   thyrochondrotomy (thyro/chondr/otomy) — surgical incision of the thyroid cartilage
   thyrooncus (thyro/oncus) — tumor of the thyroid; goiter
   parathyroid (para/thyroid) — (1) situated beside the thyroid gland; (2) any one of four small glands near the lateral lobes of the thyroid

tri-   three

Having, combining, or involving three; triply, in three ways or directions; three times; every three, every third

Examples:
   trifurcation (tri/furc/ation) — division into three parts; literally "three forks"
   trilateral (tri/later/al) — pertaining to or having three sides
   trilobate (tri/lob/ate) — having three lobes
   tripod (tri/pod) — having three feet
   triorchidism (tri/orchid/ism) — the condition of having three testes or testicles
   triplegia (tri/plegia) — paralysis of three of the extremities

ureter   ureter

A tube that carries urine from the kidney to the bladder. Note the important root **ur-** which is contained in both ureter and urethra and means urine, that is, the yellowish liquid waste product secreted by the kidneys.

Examples:
   ureteric, ureteral (ureter/ic, ureter/al) — pertaining to the ureter

Lesson 12 — Reading Assignment

ureterectasis (ureter/ectasis) — distention of the ureter

ureterocutaneostomy (ureter/o/cutan/e/ostomy) — surgical creation of an opening of the ureter on the skin, permitting drainage of urine directly to the exterior of the body

ureterolithotomy (ureter/o/lith/otomy) — the removal of a calculus (stone) from the ureter by incision

urethra   urethra

The canal through which urine is discharged from the bladder to the outside; in the male, semen is also discharged through the urethra.

Examples:

urethral (urethr/al) — pertaining to the urethra

urethrocele (urethr/o/cele) — prolapse (hernia) of the female urethra

urethroplasty (urethr/o/plast/y) — plastic surgery of the urethra; operative repair of a wound or defect in the urethra

urethrostenosis (urethr/o/sten/osis) — narrowing of the urethra

urethrostomy (urethr/o/stomy) — the formation of a permanent surgical opening into the urethra

utero-   uterus

The uterus, the hollow, muscular organ in the female which serves to protect and nourish the developing embryo and fetus during pregnancy has already been discussed under hyster- (Lesson 2) and metr- (Lesson 10); also commonly called the womb.

Note: The human organism up to the third month following pregnancy is called an embryo; thereafter, that is, the following six months until birth, it is called a fetus. Both the embryonic and fetal development take place in the uterus (see blast- in reading assignment of Lesson 14).

Examples:

uterolith (uter/o/lith) — a uterine calculus or stone

uterovesical (uter/o/vesic/al) — pertaining to the uterus and the bladder

uteropexy (uter/o/pexy) — the fixation of a displaced uterus; hysteropexy

uteritis (uter/itis) — inflammation of the uterus; metritis

vena-   vein

Any blood vessel that carries blood from some part of the body back toward the heart. This word is used together with a following descriptive word to name the many veins of the body. For diseases, abnormalities and therapeutic procedures, the rooth **phleb-** is used.

Lesson 12 — Element Recognition Exercise

Separate the elements, connecting vowels, and word terminals of the following medical words by inserting a slash mark (/) between them.

Example: thyrochondrotomy — thyro/chondr/otomy

arteriosclerosis

appendicolithiasis

thyroaplasia

splenocele

ovariorrhexis

adrenomegaly

basicranial

pelvospondylitis

venectasia

urethrocystitis

uteroplasty

sacrarthrogenic

pharyngoplegia

duodenocholedochotomy

ureteronephrectomy

laryngocentesis

bronchopneumopathy

colostomy

esophagocologastrostomy

biramous

tridactylism

ileoileostomy

iliocostal

thermotherapy

sacrolumbar

pharyngocele

ureterostenosis

laryngorhinology

basilateral

pelvitherm

urethrorrhaphy

uterolith

bronchophony

esophagomycosis

tricheiria

ileocolotomy

cryotherapy

iliolumbar

arteriostrepsis

thyroptosis

splenomyelomalacia

ovariosalpingecto my

PART II
DISEASES AND OPERATIONS
OF THE MAJOR BODY SYSTEMS
Lesson II-1 — Review

ELEMENT	AUDIONYM	VISUAL IMAGE	MEANING
ventr-	vent	See the **vent** filled with the **front** of a man!	front
vert-	vertebrae	See the **vert**ebrae that **turn**s and **turn**s!	turn
eu-	ukulele	See the **u**kulele being eaten because it is so **good**!	good
ambi-	amp, bee	See the **amp** with a **bee** on it. The **bee** is holding a phone **booth**!	both
amphi-	amp, feet	See the **amp** with **fee**t which are **round** on **both sides**!	around, on both sides
brachy-	brake	See the **brake** wearing a pair of **shorts**!	short
capit-	cap	See the **cap** with a **head** sticking through the top of it!	head
cau-	cough	See the man **cou**ghing as he reads a book. His **cou**gh **burn**s a hole right through the book!	burn
clas-	class	See the **clas**s (of students) that **break**s in half!	break
duct-	duck	See the **duc**k with an inner **tube** around its neck!	tube
fiss-	fish	See the **fis**h being **split**!	split

158

Lesson II-1 — Review

ELEMENT	AUDIONYM	VISUAL IMAGE	MEANING
ger-	jar	See the **jar** with an **old** man in it!	old
heter-	header	See the **header** with an **udder** on it!	other
infer-	inn, fur	See the **inn, fur** (an **inn** made of **fur**) **under** water!	under
hom-	home	See the **hom**e change into many **hom**es which look the **same**!	same
olfact-	oil factory	See the **oil fact**ory with a terrible **smell**!	smell
orth-	Orthodox church	See the **Orth**odox church with workers trying to make it **straight**!	straight
gyn-	gun, gin	See the **gun** shaped like a bottle of **gin** with a **female** coming out of it!	female
pachy-	pack	See the **pack** on the person's back become very **thick**!	thick
phrag-	fur rag	See the **fur rag** with the **fence**!	fence
poster-	poster	See the **poster** with people looking at the **back part** of it!	back part
cata-	catalog	See the **cata**log with **down** all over it!	down
platy-	plate	See the **plate** so **flat** all the food slides off it!	flat
pseud-	suit	See the **suit** with **false** teeth on it!	false
schiz-	skis	See the **skis** that **split**!	split

159

Lesson II-1 — Worksheet

Complete the following:

ELEMENT	AUDIONYM	MEANING
ger-	_____	_____
capit-	_____	_____
ventr-	_____	_____
cau-	_____	_____
vert-	_____	_____
clas-	_____	_____
eu-	_____	_____
fiss-	_____	_____
ambi-	_____	_____
brachy-	_____	_____
amphi-	_____	_____
duct-	_____	_____
heter-	_____	_____
poster-	_____	_____
gyn-	_____	_____
hom-	_____	_____
cata-	_____	_____
schiz-	_____	_____
olfact-	_____	_____
pseud-	_____	_____
infer-	_____	_____
pachy-	_____	_____
phrag-	_____	_____
platy-	_____	_____
orth-	_____	_____

Lesson II-1 — Reading Assignment

ambi-, ambo-   sometimes amb-, am-, an-   both, on both sides, around

You may know that ambi/dextrous means equal ease in using both hands. If you know that an intro/vert (inner turning) is a person whose thoughts and concerns are directed mostly within himself; that an extrovert (outer turning) is a person whose thoughts and concerns are directed principally toward others, then it would follow that an ambi/vert would have both "inner turning" and "outer turning" characteristics.

Examples:
   ambi/sexual — pertaining to or affecting both sexes
   ambi/ent — surrounding, on both or all sides
   am/plex/ation — braid or weave around

amphi-, ampho-   both, in two ways; roundabout, around

An amphi/theater is an oval or U-shaped structure surrounded by rows of seats. An amphi/bi/an can maintain life (bi-, bio-) in two environments. Some frogs and snakes are equally at home on water or land and are classified as amphi/bi/ans. Aircraft and tanks or other vehicles which can travel on either land or water are called amphi/bi/ans.

Examples:
   amphi/cran/ia — pain on both sides of the head
   amph/o/dipl/op/ia — double vision in both eyes

brachy-   short
   brachy/meta- — measurably short
   brachy/faci/al — low, broad face
   brachy/gnath/ia — abnormal shortness of the underjaw
   brachy/cheil/ia — shortness of the lip
   brachy/morph/ic — built along lines that are shorter than those of the normal figure
   brachy/metr/op/ia — nearsightedness

capit- (cep-, cip-)   head

You learned in Lesson 3 that cephal- means "head". Capit-, sometimes abbreviated to cep- or cip- also means "head". You may recognize the figurative use of capit- in capit/al "pertaining to the head". In the case of capit/al we mean the "head of government".

Examples:
   de/capit/ate — "head from"; the act of beheading
   oc/cipit/al — "back of head"; pertaining to the back of the head
   oc/cipit/al bone — the bone that forms the back of the skull
   bi/cep/s — "two-headed"; a muscle having two heads or points of origin; especially the large
      muscle in the front of the upper arm or the corresponding muscle at the back of the thigh

cata-, cath-, (kath-)   down, under, lower; complete

A cata/stroph/e is a complete failure or extreme "downturning". A cate/gory is lower or less than the whole. A cata/log is a complete written list.

Examples:
   cata/rrh — (rrh is an abbreviated form of rrhe-) a "flowing down"; inflammation of a mucous
      membrane with a discharge of mucus
   cata/lys/t — a "loosening down"; a substance which speeds up, or sometimes slows down, the
      rate of a chemical reaction
   cath/et/er — a "sending down"; a slender tube which is inserted into a body cavity

Lesson II-1 — Reading Assignment

cau-, caus-, caut-, caust-,   burn, burning heat
   cauter-   a searing or burning, such as with a hot iron

You may know that lye, sulphuric acid, or other chemicals which destroy or eat away are called caust/ic substances. Or perhaps you have heard someone described as having a caust/ic wit, that is, a "burning" or destructive manner of commenting.

Examples:
   caust/ic — burning or corrosive; destructive to human tissue
   caus/alg/ia — a burning pain
   cauter/ize — the application of a caust/ic substance, a hot iron, an electric current, or other
      means of killing tissue
   therm/o/cauter/y — cauter/ization by means of a heated wire or point

clas-, clad-   break, destroy

-cla/sis   the surgical procedure whereby a part, usually a bone, is broken (fractured) or rebroken (refractured) for the purpose of repair or reconstruction

Examples:
   oste/o/cla/sis — the breaking of a bone to correct a deformity
   oste/o/clast — an instrument used to perform oste/o/cla/sis
   cardi/o/cla/sis — literally a "broken heart"; actually, rupture of the heart
   dia/cla/sis — a fracture (break through or apart), especially one for a surgical purpose

duct-   a tube, a channel or canal through which a gas or liquid moves, also, "duct-" means to lead or draw.

In your home you may have a heating duct which is a tube that carries heated air from the furnace to each room. An aqueduct is a tube or channel that carries water. An orchestra con/duct/or or a tour con/duct/or is a leader. An ab/duct/or is one who leads or draws (actually forces) another away.

Examples:
   ab/duct — to draw away from the midline of the body; an instance would be the raising of the arm
      outward and to the side.
      ab/duct/or — a muscle that draws a part of the body away from the midline
      ad/duct/or — the opposite of ab/duct/or; a muscle that draws a part of the body toward the
         midline

   duct/less glands — glands producing internal secretions that are introduced directly into the
      bloodstream (rather than through a duct) for transport to the rest of the body;
      end/o/crin/e gland — the thyroid, adrenal, and pituitary glands are end/o/crin/e/s or duct/less

eu-   good, well; normal; easy

You may be familiar with a eu/log/y, "good speaking," a formal speech praising a person who has recently died; eu/thanas/ia, "good death" (thanas- is an element meaning death), which has been advocated by some as a way to deal with persons dying of incurable, painful diseases.

Examples:
   The element eu- is used in medical terms to indicate normal functioning in the form eu/ ____ /ia:

   eu/chol/ia — normal bile
   eu/glyc/em/ia — normal level of glucose in the blood

eu/kines/ia — normal movement
eu/pne/a — normal breathing, normal respiration

fiss-, fid-   to split, cleave

Nuclear fiss/ion, the splitting of atomic particles to produce nuclear energy, is currently a matter of great public concern.

Examples:
  fiss/ure — any cleft or groove, normal or otherwise
  fiss/ion — a splitting apart; a division into parts
  fiss/ul/a — a little cleft
  fiss/ura — a general term for a cleft or groove; used in anatomical nomenclature to designate the major fiss/ure/s of the body

ger-, geron-, geront-   old (in the sense of old age or an old person)

Examples:
  acr/o/ger/ia — "old extremities"; condition of premature aging of the skin of the hands and feet
  ger/iatr/ics — the branch of medicine that deals with the diseases and hygiene of old age
  geront/ology — the scientific study of the process of aging and the problems of aged people

gyn-, gynec-   female, woman

We're familiar with mono/gamy (-gamy means marriage) as meaning being married to only one person at a time and poly/gamy as meaning being married to many (that is, more than one) persons at one time. Mono/gyn/y means being married to one woman at a time; poly/gyn/y means being married to many women at one time.

Examples:
  gynec/ology — the branch of medicine dealing with the specific functions and diseases of women. The specialist is a gynec/ologist
  gynec/oid — "female-like"; of or characteristic of a woman or women
  gynec/o/mast/ia — "woman-breasted condition"; excessive development of the male mammary glands

heter-, hetero-, (-eter-)   other, different from (opposite of homo-)

To be heter/o/sexual is to have sexual interest in those of the opposite sex

Examples:
  heter/o/gen/ous — differing or opposite in structure, quality, etc.
  myel/eter/osis — morbid alteration of the spinal cord
  heter/o/top/ia — "different place"; displacement or misplacement of parts or organs

hom-, -om-, homo-, home/o/-   same, the same, equal; like, resembling (as opposed to heter- "different")

Note: The word homo also refers to the biological class which includes modern man, as well as man-like mammals such as apes and monkeys; within this class modern man is further classified as homo sapiens, "the wise one".

A homo/sexual is one who has a sexual preference for those of the same sex. Homo/gen/ized milk has been processed so that cream (the fat element) is so finely divided and emulsified as not to separate.

Lesson II-1 — Reading Assignment

Examples:
 home/o/stas/is — "standing the same"; a tendency toward uniformity or stability in the normal body states
 home/o/trans/plant — a piece of tissue taken from one individual and transplanted in another individual of the same species
 homo/hem/o/therapy — treatment by the injection of blood from another individual of the same species

infer- below
 infer/o/- below and. . .

We have a sense of the meaning "lower" or "below" in our use of the word "infer/ior."

Examples:
 infer/ior — situated below or located downward
 infer/o/later/al — situated below and to one side
 infer/o/med/ian — situated in the middle of the underside
 infer/o/poster/ior — situated below and behind

olfact- smell; to smell

Examples:
 olfact/ion — the act of smelling; the sense of smell
 olfact/o/phob/ia — morbid aversion to odors
 olfact/ory — pertaining to the sense of smell

orth- straight; correct, normal

The applications of orth- in medical terms are related to our common usage of the word "straight." Straight can be used in the sense of the same direction throughout, as in "a straight line." In expressions such as "going straight" and "straighten out" we are using "straight" in the sense of "normal" or "correct." Most medical terms using ortho- carry the meaning "correction of deformity" or "correction of malfunction."

Examples:
 orth/odont/ics — the branch of dentistry concerned with correcting and preventing irregularities of the teeth and poor "bite"
 orth/o/ped/ics — the branch of surgery dealing with the treatment of deformities, diseases, and injuries of the bones, joints, muscles, etc. (ped- refers to child since many deformities and malfunctions are con/genit/al, "born together"; that is, existing at birth; however, orth/o/ped/ics — is not confined to children.)
 an/orth/op/ia — "not straight vision"; distorted vision
 orth/osis — the straightening of a distorted part

pachy- thick

Have you ever heard an elephant referred to as a pachy/derm? Actually, any large, thick-skinned animal such as an elephant, a rhinoceros, or a hippopotamus is a pachy/derm.

Examples:
 pachy/. . ./ia — a condition of thickness
  pachy/derm/ia — skin thickness; abnormal thickness of the skin
  pachy/em/ia — blood thickness; thickening of the blood
 acr/o/pach/y — clubbed (thickened) fingers and toes

Lesson II-1 — Reading Assignment

phrag-, phrax-   to fence in, wall off, block up

Examples:
   dia/phrag/m — "blocking across"; a partition; the partition of muscles and tendons between the chest cavity and the abdominal cavity; the midriff
   urethr/o/phrax/is — blocking (obstruction) of the urethra
   kata/phrax/is — the operation to enclose or surround an organ with metal supports (a fencing in) to keep it in place

platy-   broad, flat
plak-, plax-, plat-   flat or broad like a plate; a patch of eruption

We use plate, platform, plane, platter (not only as a utensil but to describe a phonograph record). All of these words contain the impression of flatness. A plain (as in the Great Plains) carries the idea of breadth and flatness.

Examples:

   The form platy/ ___ /ia or platy/ ___ /ic — is used to describe broadness or flatness in many body parts, platy/pod/ia — flatfooted; abnormal flatness of the feet

   The form -plak/ia — indicates abnormal patches, as on the skin, mucous membrane, etc.

      leuk/o/plak/ia — the development of white patches upon the tissues of the mouth
      malac/o/plak/ia — the formation of soft patches on mucous membranes such as those of the bladder and ureters

poster-   back part, behind

Note: As you probably suspect, this element is related to the element "post-" meaning after or behind

Examples:
   poster/ior — at or toward the rear; dors/al
   poster/o/- — behind and. . .; situated behind and. . .
      poster/o/infer/ior — behind and below
      poster/o/super/ior — behind and above
      poster/o/later/al — behind and to one side

pseud-   false, imaginary; like in appearance but unlike in structure or function

You may know that a pseud/o/nym is a "false name," that is, a fictitious name or pen name used by an author who does not want his real name to be known. In medical terms pseud- is used to indicate something which looks like or has the outward appearance of one thing but, in basic structure or the way it performs, it is not the thing it appears to be.

Examples:
   pseud/o/pregnancy — false pregnancy

   The root may appear in the form pseud/. . ./ia or pseud/. . ./osis, indicating symptoms characteristic of one condition, but actually arising from some other (frequently less serious) cause

      pseud/o/esthes/ia — "false feeling"; sensations which are felt without the usual accompanying causes or stimulus
      pseud/o/cirrh/osis — apparent cirrh/osis of the liver due to some other cause

Lesson II-1 — Reading Assignment

pseud/o/ ____ /itis — "false inflammation"
pseud/o/ ____ /oma — "false tumor"

schiz- (schis-)   split

Examples:
schiz/o/phren/ia — "split mind"; a major mental disorder typically characterized by a separation (split) between the thought processes and the emotions
cheil/o/schis/is — "split lip"; harelip
schiz/onych/ia — splitting of the nails

ventr-   front. Also, belly, abdomen, cavity

Examples:
ventr/al — the front of the body; the belly side; the abdominal region; opposed to dors/al
ventr/icle — "little cavity"; small cavities or pouches; the heart ventr/icles are the lowermost heart chambers
ventro/o/- — the belly or front and. . .; the front part of. . .
ventr/o/dors/ad — from the ventr/al (front) toward the dors/al (back)
ventr/o/cyst/o/rrhaphy — the stitching (suturing) of a cyst; or the stitching of the bladder to the abdominal wall

vert-, vers-   to turn, a turn

Examples:
vert/ebra — any of the single bones or segments of the spinal column; the arrangement of bones which permits us to turn or twist our bodies
vers/ion — a displacement (turning) of the uterus; also, the operation of turning the fetus during childbirth
vert/igo — a sensation of dizziness in which we feel that we or our surrounding is turning or whirling about in a sickening manner
trans/vers/e — "turned across"; placed crosswise; situated at a right angle to the long axis of a body or organ
retro/vers/ion — "turned back"; the tipping of an entire organ backward

Lesson II-1 — Element Recognition Exercise

Separate the elements, connecting vowels, and word terminals of the following medical words by inserting a slash mark (/) between them.

ambilateral

amphicarcinogenic

brachycephalic

capitate

cataplasia

diaclasia

ductal

euesthesia

subfissure

geroderma

gynopathy

heterodont

homodont

inferior

olfactology

orthodontics

pachyderm

diaphragm

platypodia

posterior

pseudoesthesia

schizophrenia

ventral

invert

Lesson 11-2 — Review

ELEMENT	AUDIONYM	VISUAL IMAGE	MEANING
proxim-	peroxide	See the **peroxi**de with a **knee** sticking out of it! The **knee** has **rust** all over it!	nearest
scol-	school	See the **sch**ool that is **curved**!	curved
apo-	apple	See the **ap**ple running **away from** you!	away from
di-	dye	See the **dye** coming out both ends of the bottle to **dye** material **twice**!	twice
dia-	diet pill	See the **dia**t pill with a hand stuck **through** it!	through
eury-	urinal	See the **uri**nal that became very **broad**!	broad
pect-	pecked	See the tree that has been **pecked**. It has a treasure **chest** in it!	chest
necr-	neck	See the **nec**k with a **dead** fish around it!	dead
mi-	mice	See the **mi**ce taking a **less**on on the piano!	less
morph-	mower roof	See the **mo**wer with a **r**oof. It has **forms** flying out of it!	form
dis-	discus	See the **dis**cus falling **apart**!	apart
fac-	factory	See the **fac**tory that **makes dew** drops!	make, do
lept-	leopard	See the **lep**oard that is very **slender**!	slender

Lesson 11-2 — Review

ELEMENT	AUDIONYM	VISUAL IMAGE	MEANING
lymph-	limp	See the person **limp**ing because he has **water** and **fluid** strapped to his leg!	watery fluid
meta-	metal cabinet	See the **meta**l cabinet with a **bee yawn**ing inside it!	beyond
-rrhag	raging river	See the **rag**ing river and the balloons **burst**ing with **fort**s inside them!	burst, burst forth
sta-	stand	See the music **sta**nd with another **sta**nd on top of it!	stand
ton-	ton	See the **ton** (truck) being **stretched**!	stretch
volv-	valve	See the **valv**e with **tea roll**s coming out of it!	to roll
splanchn-	"S" plank	See the **"S" plank** with an **inner tube** and **organs** on it!	internal organs
-rrhe	reed instrument	See the **ree**d instrument with something **flow**ing out of it!	flow
med-	meat	See the **meat** with a hole in the **middle** of it!	middle
xer-	zero	See the **zer**o on the thermometer with the clothes **dry**er bursting out of it!	dry
per-	purr	See the cat that **purr**s and then **throws out** the whole family! **Throw out - throughout**.	throughout
blast-	blast	See the space ship **blast**ing off. It turns into a **bud**!	bud

169

Lesson II-2 — Worksheet

Complete the following:

ELEMENT	AUDIONYM	MEANING
xer-		
sta-		
proxim-		
morph-		
necr-		
dia-		
di-		
fac-		
pect-		
lymph-		
ton-		
-rrhe		
per-		
volv-		
lept-		
blast-		
meta-		
apo-		
mi-		
scol-		
eury-		
dis-		
med-		
-rrhag		
splanchn-		

Lesson II-2 — Reading Assignment

apo-   away from, separation, from; lack

To apo/log/ize is to "speak away." Figuratively we "speak away" or say something which corrects some previous action or words which have given offense to someone.

Examples:
    apo/phy/sis — a "growth away from"; an outgrowth, especially a bony outgrowth
    apo/gen/y — lack of the power to reproduce

blast-   bud, shoot, sprout, embry/onic cell

The root "blast-" indicates a relationship to something which is formative on the order of a sprouting seed; more specifically to an embry/o. You probably know that a human in the mother's womb is called an embry/o. Technically, the human organism in the mother's womb is called an embry/o during the early stages of pregnancy: the period from one week after conception to the end of the second month. From the third month on it is called a fet/us. In its early stages (about the first week or so) the embry/o consists of increasing layers of cells around a central cavity somewhat in the shape of a hollow sphere. At this stage it is called a blast/ul/a (a little bud).

Examples:
    blast (or as word ending -blast) — an immature (lacking complete development) stage in cell
        development; a stage in which the final characteristics of the cell are not yet apparent
    angi/o/blast (also called angi/o/derm) — the formative tissue from which blood cells are formed
    blast/oma — a tumor formed from tissues the same as those in the location in which it arises, as
        contrasted to a tumor composed of tissues in addition to or other than those in the area from
        which it develops
    angi/o/blast/oma — a blood vessel tumor
    lip/o/blast — a tissue cell which develops into a fat cell; an embry/onic fat cell
    lip/o/blast/oma — a tumor made up of lip/o/blast/s or embry/onic fat cells

di-   twice, double, twofold

Di/ox/ide/s (such as carbon di/ox/ide) are oxides containing two atoms of oxygen for each molecule

Examples:
    di/morph/ic — "double form"; occurring in two distinct forms
    di/gloss/ia — double tongue
    di/hyster/ia — condition of having a double uterus

dia-   across, through, apart

Dia/meter is a straight line passing through a circle, or the measure of such a line.

Examples:
    dia/rrhe/a — a "flowing through"; an excessive flow of loose matter from the bowels
    dia/lys/is — a "loosening apart"; a process by which substances in solution are separated from
        each other; especially the separation of impurities from the blood during kidney failure
    dia/phrag/m — a "wall across"; a membrane across the body separating the chest from the
        abdomen

dis-   apart, away, asunder; opposite of

This prefix is similar to de- and is widely used both in medicine and in common English. Sometimes it can mean so far apart as to be the opposite of:
    dis/ease — the opposite of being at ease; "not ease"
    dis/able — the opposite of being able; "not able"

Lesson II-2 — Reading Assignment

Sometimes it can mean separation, a "putting away":
   dis/miss — a dis/miss/al (particularly from a job) is a separation

Examples:
   dis/sect — "cut apart"; that is, to cut in many pieces
   dis/loc/ation — "apart or away from its place"; specifically, to dis/place a bone from its correct loc/ation
   dis/esthes/ia — the "opposite feeling"; dis/comfort

eury-   wide, broad (opposed to sten- narrow)

Since the effect of widening or broadening is to increase in size, eury- carries the meaning "enlargement" due to widening or broadening

Examples:
   an/eury/sm — (frequently changed to an/eur/ism) a sac formed by the local enlargement of the weakened wall of an artery, caused by disease or injury
   proct/eury/sis — dilatation (widening) of the rectum by an instrument
   eury/cephal/ous — having a wide head

fac-, fact-, fic-, fect-   to do, make, cause
fac-, faci-, fici-   face; outer surface; form, figure

We have chosen to discuss these two elements together because of their similarity and because of the wide usage that each has.

You are familiar with a faci/al as a treatment intended to improve the skin of the face. A fac/ade is the front part of anything, the outer surface. Super/fici/al means of or being on the surface; sometimes used figuratively to mean shallow in the sense of the obvious and easily seen rather than the deep and profound.

You are also familiar with a factory in which things are manu/fact/ured. (manu- means "hand" as in manu/al training; manu/al labor. Manu/fact/ure originally meant "made by hand" although it has now been extended to mean things made by machinery.) To fac/il/it/ate is to make easy. The fac/ul/ty of the schools you have attended or are attending is provided to make or cause easy learning, or, as easy as the subject matter and the student permit. In fac/il/it/at/ing the learning process the fac/ul/ty presents fact/s (that which was done). A good instructor is both ef/fect/ive and ef/fici/ent.

lept-   thin, slender, delicate (literally a peel)

Examples:
   lept/o/chym/ia — thinness (meagerness) of body fluids
   lept/o/dactyl/y — abnormal slenderness of fingers and toes
   lept/o/dermic — thin skinned

lymph-   watery fluid

One of the major fluids of the body found in all parts of the body. Other major fluids are blood and tissue fluid. Lymph is a pale fluid that bathes the tissues, passes into lymph channels and ducts, and is discharged into the blood.

Examples:
   lymph/aden — a combination of elements referring to a lymph gland or lymph node.

   Note: The names "lymph gland" and "lymph node" are synonyms. "Lymph node" is the preferred name although "lymph gland" is widely used.

Lesson II-2 — Reading Assignment

"node" means "knot"; a knotty swelling or protuberance (A protuberance is something which bulges or sticks out.)

med-, mes, medi-, mesi- middle, intermediate

You may know that a medi/al strip on a highway is a strip down the middle; that an inter/medi/ary is one who comes in between (that is, takes a middle position) without bias toward either side. In non-medical English we are inclined to use the prefix med- or mid- more frequently to designate a middle, the middle, something in between. In medical terminology mes- is the more frequently used prefix.

Examples:
mes/enter/y — a membranous fold attaching the small intestine to the base of the abdominal wall
mes/o/nas/al — situated in the middle of the nose
mes/o/derm — the middle layer of cells in an embryo from which the skeletal, reproductive, muscular, vascular, connective, etc. tissues develop. Logically enough, the ecto/derm is the outside layer and the endo/derm is the inside layer
mediastin/um — "occurring in the middle"; a membranous partition between two cavities of the body; especially the membrane separating the lungs

meta- beyond, change, transformation; after

Examples:
meta/bol/ism — (bol- means to throw) to "throw beyond"; change; all of the physical and chemical changes and processes continuously going on in the body by which growth is achieved and energy released
meta/morph/o/sis — "form change"; change in shape or structure
meta/sta/sis — a "change in standing or status"; the spread of disease from one part of the body to another
meta/plas/ia — "development change"; abnormal change of one type of tissue to another; also, conversion of one tissue into another, as the cartilage of the infant into the bone of the adult

mio-, meio- less, smaller

We commonly use a variation of this element in the form min-. Min/or means lesser in size, amount, number, extent, importance, etc. To di/min/ish is to make less. In subtraction, four min/us two means that four is to be diminished (that is, made less or smaller) by two.

Examples:
-mio/sis, -mei/osis — condition of decrease; disintegration
oste/o/mio/sis — "bone lessening"; disintegration of a bone
rhin/o/mio/sis — "nose lessening"; surgery for the reduction of the size of the nose
mio/cardia — the contraction (squeezing thus lessening) movement of the heart; also called systole

morph- form, shape, figure

Examples:
-morph/ic, -morph/ous — having a (specified) shape
mono/morph/ous — "single shape"; existing in one form only; having the same form throughout all stages of development
iso/morph/ic — "equal shape"; having similar or identical structure or form
a/morph/ous — "no shape"; without definite form; shapeless
meta/morph/osis — change in form, shape, structure, or substance

Lesson II-2 — Reading Assignment

necr-   dead

  Examples:
  necr/osis — death of tissue
  -necr/o/sis — condition of dead tissue
    rhin/o/necr/osis — necr/osis of the nasal bones
    oste/o/necr/osis — necr/osis of a bone
  necr/ectomy — the cutting away (excision) of dead material
  necr/ology — statistics or records of death

pect-, pector-   the chest, thorax; the part of the body enclosed by the ribs

  Examples:
  ex/pector/ate — "out of the chest"; to cough and spit out (phlegm, mucus, etc.)
  pector/algia — pain in the chest
  angina pector/is — (angina means a choking, a strangling) pain in the chest, sometimes extend-
    ing to the left arm, caused by a sudden decrease of the blood supply to the heart muscle

per-   throughout, through; thoroughly, excessively

  Examples:
  per/acute — excessively acute or sharp
  per/nas/al — "through the nose"; performed through the nose
  per/cutan/eous — "through the skin"; performed through the skin as an injection

proxim-   near, nearest

  We can describe locations as being "in the proxim/ity of. . ." by which we mean "near" or "close to."
  An ap/proxim/ation is an estimate, something which is close (near) enough for practical purposes.

  Examples:
  proxim/al — nearest; closer to any point of reference; opposed to dist/al (farthest)
  proxim/ate — next or nearest
  proxim/ad — toward the proxim/al (nearest) end

-rrhag- (rhag-)   burst forth; burst

  -rrhag/ia — usually a bursting forth of blood; heavy bleeding

  Examples:
  hem/o/rrhag/e — (shortened from hem/o/rrhag/ia) a substantial flow of blood; bleeding

    Hem/o/rrhag/e fully carries the meaning "blood flow" since it contains the root hem-. However,
      the appearance of the ending -rrhag/ia usually carries the meaning "blood flow" from the
      body part to which it is attached
    enter/o/rrhag/ia — intestinal blood flow
    metr/o/rrhag/ia — uterine bleeding
    odont/o/rrhag/ia — "tooth bleeding"
    hem/o/rrhag/e — profuse bleeding e.g., following the extraction of teeth

Lesson II-2 — Reading Assignment

-rrhe- (rhe-)   to flow

Examples:
   dia/rrhe/a — "to flow through"; excessive looseness or frequency of bowel movements
   ot/o/rrhe/a — "ear flow"; a discharge from the ear
   rhe/um — any watery or cata/rrh/al discharge
   cata/rrh — "flow down," shortened from cata/rrhe; inflammation of mucous membrane with a
      free discharge of mucus; runny (that is, flowing) nose

scol-, scoli-   curved, twisted, crooked

Examples:
   -scoli/osis — condition of curvature, crookedness
   rach/i/scoli/osis — curvature of the spine; more frequently shortened to scoli/osis without the
      preceeding rachi-
   scolec- — form of scol-, denoting relationship to a worm; worm-shaped; can refer to the appen-
      dix which has the shape of a worm, as in scolec-tomy, a synonym for the preferred term
      "append/ectomy."

   Note: There are many appendixes (from ad — to + pend — hang) "hanging to" various
      body structures. The one most frequently encountered is the worm-shaped (scolec/oid)
      pouching out (di/vert/ic/ul/um) from the small intestine. Although generally called "the ap-
      pendix" its technical name is the "vermi/form (vermi- is a root also meaning "worm") (see
      Lesson 12 - appendic).

   scolec/oid — worm-shaped

splanchn-, splanchno-   internal organs, viscera, entrails; heart, liver, intestines, etc.

Examples:
   eu/splanchn/ia — a normal (good) condition of the internal organs
   splanchn/ec/top/ia — out of place internal organ
   splanchn/odyn/ia — pain in an internal organ

sta-, ste-, stas-   set, cause to stand, fix

This element carries meanings similar to those which we use in our words such as: sta/nd, sta/ble,
sta/tionary, sta/tus, sta/ck, all of which carry the idea of remaining or being in a fixed position.

Examples:
   sta/sis — a stoppage of the flow of blood or other body fluid in any body part

   -sta/sis — a stoppage, standing, arresting
      dia/sta/sis — "standing apart"; a form of bone dislocation
      meta/stasis — "standing beyond"; the traveling of a disease process from one part of the
         body to another
   -stas/ia — a condition of standing; a stoppage
      chole/stas/ia — stoppage or suppression of the flow of bile
   hem/o/sta/sis, hem/o/stas/ia — the arrest of the escape of blood; the checking of the flow of
      blood
   hem/o/stat — anything used to stop bleeding; a clamplike instrument used in surgery; a
      medicine that hastens clotting

Lesson II-2 — Reading Assignment

ton-   a stretching, tension

   tein- (tan-, ten-), tas-, tend-, tens- — to stretch, strain
   tetan- — stretched; spasm

Here is a family of elements all of which carry the idea of stretching. Our word ton/e, meaning a vocal or musical sound, originates in the noise produced by the vibrating of a stretched string. Vocal sounds are produced by the vibrating vocal cords under various stages of tens/ion or stretching. To be tens/e or under tens/ion is to be stretched, tight, strained, taut. To ex/tend is to stretch out producing an ex/tens/ion of greater or lesser ex/tent; to dis/tend is to stretch apart producing a dis/tens/ion.

Examples:
   ton/e — the normal degree of vigor and tens/ion; in muscle, the resistance to stretching when in a relaxed state
   ton/ic — producing and restoring the normal tone
   a/ton/y — "not tone"; lack of tone
   tetan/us — lockjaw; an acute infectious disease characterized by spasmodic contractions and rigidity of some or all of the voluntary muscles
   bronch/o/tetan/y — bronch/o/spasm; contraction of the bronchial tubes due to excessive constriction of the muscles surrounding them
   -ec/tas/y — a stretching; the act of stretching
   lith/ec/tas/y — removal of a stone through the stretched urethra

volv-   to turn, roll, roll over; a turning or rolling
   volut- — a turning or rolling motion

To re/volve is to turn back or turn again. A re/volut/ion is a rolling back of authority. To be in/volv/ed is to be rolled up in some occupation, cause or person. E/volut/ion is a "turning out," an "unfolding." Our word "volume" comes from the ancient writings in the form of scrolls which were rolled up sheets of parchment.

Examples:
   con/volut/ion — "rolled together"; a twisting, coiling or winding together; specifically, any of the folds or ridges on the surface of the brain
   volv/ul/us — intestinal obstruction due to a knotting and twisting of the bowel
      volv/ul/ate — to twist or form a knot
   in/volut/e — to return (re/turn) to normal size after enlargement
      sub/in/volut/ion — "less than re/turn"; incomplete
         in/volut/ion; failure of a part to return to its normal size and condition after enlargement

xer-   dry

Note: A Xer/ox copier is a dry copier and is in contrast to the wet copiers, such as in photographic processes which were used prior to the invention of the dry process.

Examples:
   xer/osis — abnormal dryness as of the eye or skin
   xer/o/derm/a — "dry skin"; dryness and roughness of the skin
   xer/o/cheil/ia — "dry lips"; dryness of the lips

Lesson II-2 — Element Recognition Exercise

Separate the elements, connecting vowels, and word terminals of the following medical words by inserting a slash mark (/) between them.

apogeny

blastoma

dimorphic

diameter

disable

eurycephalous

leptodermic

lymphadenoma

medial

metamorphosis

miocardia

monomorphous

necrectomy

pectus

pernasal

proximal

hemorrhage

diarrhea

scoliosis

splanchnodynia

hemostasis

tonic

volvulus

xerocheilia

REFERENCE SECTION AND FINAL TEST
FAMILIAR ELEMENTS

There are a number of useful medical elements imbedded in words with which you are familiar. The purpose of this section is to make you aware of these elements, to give them a medical definition, and to show you how they are related to medical terms.

abdomin- the abdomen; the belly; the part of the body, except for the back, between the thorax (chest) and the pelvis (hip area)

abdomin/al — pertaining to the abdomen
abdomin/ous — "full abdomen"; big-bellied
abdomin/algia — "belly-ache"; pain in the abdomen
abdomin/o/cardi/ac — pertaining to the abdomen and the heart

abdomin/o/hyster/ectomy — hysterectomy performed through an abdominal incision; a hysterectomy performed through the abdomen (abdominal hysterectomy), as opposed to a hysterectomy performed through the vagina (vaginal hysterectomy)

ana-, an- up, up from below

To analyze is to "loosen up", to separate (a thing, idea, etc.) into its parts. Ana/tomy is a "cutting up", the dissecting of a plant or animal in order to examine its parts. Ana/tomy, therefore, has come to be known as the science of the form and structure of plants or animals based on the "cutting up" which has been performed.

ana/stom/osis — "a state of joining up by mouths or openings"; an interconnect in between blood vessels; a surgical procedure whereby one hollow or tubular organ is joined to another

an enter/o-enter/o/stomy — is an intestinal ana/stom/osis since the term denotes the surgical procedure of forming a connection between two parts of the intestine

ana/plast/ic — "forming back"; restoring a lost or missing part
ana/plast/y — restorative or plastic surgery

bio- (bi-) life

You have seen this root in:
Bio/logy — "life science"; the science that deals with living matter

bio/graph/y — "life writing"; written history of a person's life

Medical applications include:
bi/ops/y — "appearance of life" (ops- look, appearance, view; related to op-, ops- "see"); the removal of tissues, cells, or fluids from the living body for examination or study

-bio(tic): pertaining to life
anti/bio/tic: — a substance produced by a microorganism (such as bacteria) having the capacity to inhibit the growth or kill another microorganism (such as a disease germ); in this sense, tending to inhibit or destroy life

brevi- short

You have seen this root in:
brevi/ty — shortness of duration; shortness of time
ab/brevi/ate — to shorten; to make brief

FAMILIAR ELEMENTS

Medical applications include:
- brevi/lingu/al — "short tongued"
- brevi/flex/or — a short flexor muscle

cav-, cavit-   hollow

This root is familiar in:
- cav/e — a hollow space inside the earth
- cavit/y — a hole or hollow place; a hollow space in a tooth especially when caused by decay; a natural hollow place within the body
- cavern — a cave, especially a large cave

The root carries medical meanings:
- cav — a small enclosed space within the body or an organ
- cavit — appearing as "cavit/y"; used to designate hollow spaces in the body and lesions of a tooth produced by dental caries
- cavern — the general element used to designate a cavity

Examples:
- cavern/o/scop/y — inspection of the cavities of the lung by means of an instrument
- con/cave — "very hollow"; hollow and curved like the inside half of a hollow ball
- cavern/ous — "full of caves"; containing caverns or hollow spaces

circum-   around

This prefix is familiar in:
- circum/ference — the line forming the boundary of ("surrounding") a circle
- circum/stantial — as in "circumstantial evidence" or in the phrase "depending on the circumstances." In both of these phrases the circum- root carries the meaning of "surrounding" or "around."

The same idea of "around," "about," "on all sides" applies to medical words
- circum/or/al — around or near the mouth
- circum/ren/al — around or near the kidney
- circum/duct/ion — "draw around"; the circular movement of a limb or of an eye

com-, con-   with, together, completely

To com/press is to press together. Con/centr/ic circles are circles having the same center or having a center "together" with each other

dist-   far

Familiar in:
- dist/ant, dist/ance, out/dist/ance, all of which carry the meanings of "far," "away from."

Medical term:
- dist/al — remote; farther from any point of reference

EENT: used to designate ear, eyes, nose, throat. This is an acronym (recall acr- meaning "tip, extremity" and -nym as in audi/o/nym meaning "name"). An acronym is a word formed from the first letters of a series of words; in this case (E)ar, (E)ye, (N)ose, (T)hroat. Although EENT is not a technical medical word it is commonly used to designate the area of practice of a doctor specializing in ear, eye, nose, and throat disease and conditions.

FAMILIAR ELEMENTS

en-, em-   in, within, into (same as in-)

To en/close is to close in. To em/brace is to fold in, to hug

fibr-   fiber, filament

A fiber is a slender threadlike structure. We recognize the word as it applies to textiles such as wool fibers, cotton fibers, nylon fibers, etc. Our bodies contain structures which are made up of similar long threadlike strands. Nerves and muscles are notable examples. Tumors may consist either partially or entirely of fibr/ous contents.

Examples:
   fibr/il — a very small fiber
   fibr/oma — a tumor composed mainly of fibr/ous tissue
   lip/o/fibr/oma — a fibr/oma containing fatty elements
   fibr/o/muscul/ar — composed of fibr/ous and muscular tissue

flex-, flect-   to bend, turn

Did you ever flex your muscles? How many times have you seen your re/flect/ion in a mirror? Bending was involved in both cases. In the case of the mirror light was re/flect/ed or bent back toward your eyes.

Examples:
   flex/ure — a bending; a bent portion of a structure or organ
   circum/flex — "bent around"; curved like a bow; a structure which has the form of a bent bow
   retro/flex/ion — "bending backward"; the bending of an organ so that its top is turned backward; essentially, a U-shape.

in-   (also il-, im-, ir-) not

As used in incapable, illogical, impossible, irregular

infer-   below
infero-   below and. . .; on the underside and. . .

We can readily recognize the meanings "below" or "under" or "lower" in the words infer/ior and infer/ior/ity. In our ordinary usage the meaning is figurative in the sense that achievement, status, quality, etc., are lower than or under or below some acceptable standard. Infer/ior and infer/ior/ity are contrasted with super/ior and super/ior/ity

In medical terms, infer- and infero- usually mean located underneath, below, on the under side of. In medical terminology we discussed the element infra- meaning "beneath." To summarize:

   infer- almost always in the form "infer/ior," means "situated below" or "directed downward"; usually to refer to the lower surface of an organ or other structure.

   infero — is used with another word element as a directional pointer; below and. . . (See below, that is, the infer/ior part of this duscussion.)

   infra — is used with another word element, also as a direction pointer meaning situated, formed, or occurring beneath.

Examples:
   infero/later/al — situated below and to one side

FAMILIAR ELEMENTS

infero/medi/an — situated in the middle of the underside
infero/poster/ior — situated below and behind
infra/umbilic/al — beneath the navel or "belly button"

loc-   place

Loc/al means "pertaining to a place." A loc/ation is a place. To loc/ate means to find a place.

Examples:
loc/us — a place
loc/ul/us — "a small place"; a small space or cavity
loc/ul/i — "small places"; plural of luc/ul/us
dis/loc/ation — "apart from place"; the dis/place/ment of any part, more especially of a bone

mono-   one, alone, single; limited to one part

A mono-tone is one tone or a single tone. Mono/gamy means being married to only one person. A mono/plane has a single wing.

Examples:
mono/layer — consisting of a single layer
mono/pleg/ia — paralysis of a single part
mon/oste/o/tic — pertaining to or affecting a single bone

multi-   many, much; having or consisting of more than one

A multi/tude is a large number of things or persons. To multi/ply is to increase in number. Multi/colored is more than one color.

Examples:
multi/form — occurring in many forms
multi/rooted — having more than one root as the molar teeth
multi-articular — pertaining to or affecting many joints

muscul-   muscle

We readily recognize a muscul/ar person as one having well-developed or prominent muscles.
muscul/o/cut/aneous — pertaining to or supplying both muscles and skin
inter/muscul/ar — situated between muscles

narc-, narcot-   numbness, stupor, lethargy

We are very much aware of the problems caused by narcot/ics including the numbing effect which many of these substances produce. Narc/osis is the "condition of numbness" which can be produced by narcot/ics.

Examples:
electr/o/narc/osis — electroshock; unconsciousness produced by passing an electric current through the brain of a patient; used in treating some forms of mental illness
en/cephal/o/narc/osis — stupor due to brain disease
narcot/ism — addiction to narcot/ics

nas-   nose

This root is familiar in such expressions involving the nose as "nasal voice," "nasal spray," "nasal drip"

FAMILIAR ELEMENTS

Examples:
   per/nas/al — "through the nose"; performed through the nose, such as a surgical procedure or
      injection
   nas/o/pharynx — the space where the nasal passages enter the pharynx
   sub/nasal — situated below the nose

nox-, nos-   disease, illness

A nox/ious gas is one which can cause illness. An ob/nox/ious person is one who is so unpleasant
or offensive as to figuratively be "sickening."

Examples:
   -nos/is — word ending indicating disease
      troph/o/nos/is — any disease or disorder due to nutritional causes
      trich/o/nos/is — any disease of the hair
      hemat/o/nos/is — any disease of the blood

   -nos/ology — word ending denoting the classification of diseases
      nos/ology — the science of the classification of diseases
      derm/o/nos/ology — the classification of skin diseases

   nos/o/gen/ic — causing disease

palat-   palate; the roof of the mouth consisting of a hard bony forward part (the hard palate) and a
soft fleshy back part (the soft palate)

This root is familiar in the word "palat/able" by which we mean pleasant or acceptable to the taste.
We now know that the sense of taste (taste buds) is principally in the tongue. However the earlier
idea that taste arose from the roof of the mouth (the palate) persists in the word "palat/able."

Examples:
   palat/o/gloss/al — pertaining to the roof of the mouth (palate) and tongue
   trans/palat/al — performed through the roof of the mouth
   palat/o/plasty — plastic reconstruction of the palate, including cleft palate operations
   cleft palat/e — a con/genit/al deformity consisting of a fiss/ure (cleft) from front to back along the
      middle of the mouth

pelv-, pelvis   the basin-like cavity formed by the ring of bones in the lower back part of the trunk,
supporting the spinal column and resting on the legs

Most of us, having seen human skeletons or their representations, and being aware of the bony
structure of our own bodies, know that the pelvis is somewhere in the area of our hips. For the
purpose of applying medical terminology we need to know that it consists of the ring of bones forming
a basinlike structure in the area where our spinal column ends and from which our thigh bones
extend.

Examples:
   intra/pelv/ic — within the pelvis
   pelvi/meter — an instrument for measuring the diameters and space (capacity) of the pelvis
   pelvi/tomy — the operation of cutting the pelvis at any point in order to facilitate delivery

proxim-   near

We encounter proxim- in: proxim/ity, as in the sentence, "The disturbance occurred in the proximity
of (near) City Hall."

182

FAMILIAR ELEMENTS

ap/proxim/ate or ap/proxim/ate/ly, as in, "It takes approximately (nearly) three hours to go from here to there."

Medical term:
   prosim/al — nearest; closer to any point of reference

In medical descriptions major points of reference are:
   the center of the body; an imaginary line drawn from the middle of the forehead and continuing to the space between the two feet, thus dividing the body into two halves

   points of attachment such as the shoulder by which the arm is connected with the main part (or trunk) of the body

re-   back, back again; contrary, opposite

   The prefix re- appears in many words we commonly use: re/admit, re/affirm, re/appear, re/assemble, re/assign, re/awaken, re/attempt, re/authorize. Note that we have attached re- to a few words at the beginning of the alphabet. There are many more words which can be formed using re- as a prefix.

   Examples:
      re/action — opposite action, or counteraction
      re/flex — "bend back"; "bend again"; a kind of "re/action"
      re/flex action — an "automatic" response as in unthinkingly raising a hand to ward off a blow
      re/spir/ation — "breathing back"; the "back and forth" action of the lungs in inhalation and exhalation

sect- (-sect)   a cut or division; to cut or divide

   To dis/sect is to cut apart; to bi/sect is to cut in two; to inter/sect is to cut between; a sect/ion is a division or "cutting out"; a religious sect is one which has broken away ("cut out" or split away) from an established church.

   In medical terminology the meaning is practically synonymous with -otomy in designating the act, process, or product of cutting; specifically, an incision in surgery.

   Examples:
      trans/sect/ion — "cut across"; the process of cutting across or dividing by cutting
      re/sect/ion — "cut again" (in the sense of being recut or cut out); the surgical removal of part of an organ, bone, etc. Compare -ectomy, "surgical removal," with re/sect/ion, "surgical removal of part of."
      cesarean sect/ion — incision through the abdominal and uterine walls for the delivery of a fetus

skelet-, skeleton   the bony framework of the body

   The element skelet- fairly leaps out at us from the familiar words skelet/al and skelet/on

   Examples:
      skelet/al — pertaining to the bones of the body
      skelet/al system — the bones of the body acting together in their functions to provide support and give shape to the body, and, with the attached tendons, muscles, and ligaments, make body movement possible.
      end/o/skelet/al — pertaining to the bones of the body enclosed by the skin and muscles, as distinguished from exo/skelet/al
      exo/skeletal — pertaining to a hard structure developed on the outside of the body such as the shell of a crab or turtle; also applied to the hard outer structures in humans such as hair, nails, teeth, etc.

FAMILIAR ELEMENTS

super-   over, over and above (in the sense of excessive); higher in quantity, quality, or degree

Examples:
super/cili/um — "over the eyelid or eyelash"; the eyebrow
super/lethal — "excessively lethal"; more than enough to cause death
super/cerebr/al — in the upper part of the cerebrum

tors-, tort-   twist, turn

A con/tort/ion/ist is a person, usually a theatrical or circus acrobat, who can twist his body into unnatural positions. Tort/ure comes from the twisting devices used to inflict severe pain. A tort/uous road is full of twists, turns, curves, and windings. To dis/tort may be to literally twist some object out of shape or, figuratively, to twist a fact or facts.

Examples:
de/tors/ion — the correction of a curvature or deformity
tort/i/coll/is — "twisted neck" (coll- 'neck'); wry neck; a spasm or contraction of the muscles on one side of the neck, causing the head to be tilted and twisted

tox-   poison

You may know that a tox/ic substance is a substance which is poisonous. Although in/tox/ic/ation is usually associated with an excessive use of alcohol, in medicine the word means poisoning or becoming poisoned by any substance such as alcohol and other drugs, serums, acids, etc.

Examples:
tox/in — a poison; a poisonous substance usually released by bacteria
anti/toxin — "against poison"; a neutralizer of a tox/in; antibody (a counter poison) produced in the body which is capable of producing a specific immunity to a specific germ or virus
tox/em/ia — condition resulting from poisons circulating in the blood
ecto/tox/em/ia — tox/em/ia produced by a substance introduced from outside the body

ultra-   beyond, excessive

To be ultra/conservative is to be excessively conservative. To be ultra/modern is to be modern beyond the current norm. Ultra/sonic designates a frequency of mechanical vibrations beyond the range our ears can hear.

Examples:
ultra/lig/ation — ligation (tying) of a vessel beyond the point of origin of a branch
ultra/some — any body so small that it is invisible (beyond seeing) even when aided by the most powerful microscope
ultra/virus — an extremely (excessively) small disease-producing agent

vertebr-, vertebra   any of the single bones or segments of the spinal column

Here is another element which seems obvious. A vertebra or the plural vertebrae is well known from courses in biology or health which we have taken. See spondyl- in Reading Assignment of Lesson 4.

Examples:
vertebr/ate — having a spinal column or backbone; any of the animals including all mammals, fishes, birds, reptiles, and amphibians which have a spinal column
in/vertebr/ate — "not vertebr/ate"; lacking a spinal column; a division of the animal kingdom which includes all animals other than mammals, fishes, birds, reptiles, and amphibians
vertebr/arteri/al — pertaining to the vertebr/al artery (an artery carrying blood to the vertebrae)

APPLICATION OF ELEMENTS
TO SOME MEDICAL CLASSIFICATIONS

Branches of Medicine

ana/tomy: "cut up"; science of the structure of the body and relationship of its parts

embry/ology: "study of the first stages of the fertilized egg"; study of the formation and development of the embryo

hist/ology: "study of tissue"; study of the structure, composition, and function of normal cells and tissues

path/ology: "study of disease"; study of the changes in the structure or functions of the body caused by disease

physi/ology: "study of the body"; study of the normal functions and activities of the body

Major Medical Specialties and Specialists

There are corresponding endings which are used to form the words designating the specialist, the "one who", the "healer":

ist: which generally combines with:

   -olog(y) — to form -olog/ist
   -iatr(y) — to form -iatrist
   -ian — which combines with iatric(s) to form -iatrician

Two endings dominate the words designating medical specialties:

-ology: which in this application means, broadly, "study of" and, more narrowly, "science of"

-iatry or -iatrics: which carry the meaning "healing" or "treatment of disease"

an/esthes/i/ology: "science of lack of feeling"; dealing with the administration of an/esthet/ic/s to produce loss of feeling or consciousness, usually in conjunction with forms of medical treatment such as surgery

   an/esthes/i/ologist — the specialist

cardi/ology: "science of the heart"; dealing with the heart, its functions, and its diseases

   cardi/ologist — the specialist

dermat/ology: "science of the skin"; dealing with the skin and its diseases

   dermat/ologist — the specialist

ear, eye, nose, throat   (frequently referred to as EENT)

end/o/crin/ology: "science of 'secreting within' "; dealing with the end/o/crin/e glands and the internal secretions (products of the thyroid, spleen, adrenals, testicles, pituitary, etc.) of the body

   end/o/crin/ologist — the specialist

APPLICATION OF ELEMENTS
TO SOME MEDICAL CLASSIFICATIONS

Major Medical Specialties and Specialists

ger/i/atrics: "treatment of disease of old age"; dealing with the diseases and hygiene of old age

    ger/iatrician — the specialist

gynec/ology: "science of females"; dealing with the specific functions, diseases, etc. of women

    gynec/ologist — the specialist

internal medicine: dealing with the diagnosis and nonsurgical treatment of disease

    intern/ist — the specialist (**Note:** an intern is a person, generally newly graduated from medical school, serving an apprenticeship in a hospital)

laryng/ology: "science of throat"; dealing with the throat and its diseases

    laryng/ologist — the specialist

neur/o/surgery: "surgery of the nerves"; surgery involving the nervous system including the brain and spinal cord

    neur/o/surgeon — the specialist

obstetr/ics: originally derived from a term applied to a midwife literally meaning "she who stands before" (ob- before plus stetr-, a variation of **sta-** to stand); concerned with the care and treatment of women during pregnancy, childbirth, and the period immediately following

    obstetr/ician — the specialist

ophthalm/ology: "science of eye"; dealing with the structure, functions, and disorders of the eye

    ophthalm/ologist — the specialist

orth/o/ped/ics (orth/o/ped/ic surgery): "child straightening"; surgery dealing with the treatment of deformities, diseases, and injuries of bones, joints, muscles, ligaments, etc. So called because many deformities are con/genit/al and thus are discovered and corrected in childhood

    orth/o/ped/ist — the specialist (May also be called "orth/o/ped/ic surgeon" or, more briefly, "orthopod.")

ot/ology: "science of ear"; dealing with the disorders of the ear

    ot/ologist — the specialist

ped/iatrics: "science of child"; dealing with the hygienic care of children and diseases peculiar to them

    ped/iatrician — the specialist

plast/ic surgery: "reparative surgery"; surgery dealing with the repair or restoration of injured, deformed, or destroyed parts of the body, especially by transferring tissue, such as skin or bone,

Major Medical Specialties and Specialists

from other parts or from another individual

    plast/ic surgeon — the specialist

proct/ology: "science of rectum"; dealing with the rectum and anus and their diseases

    proct/ologist — the specialist

psych/iatry: "science of mind"; concerned with the study, treatment, and prevention of disorders of the mind

    psych/iatrist — the specialist

radi/ology: "science of rays"; dealing with X-rays and other forms of radiant energy for X-raying body parts and treating diseases

    radi/ologist — the specialist

rhin/ology: "science of nose"; dealing with the nose and its diseases

    rhin/ologist — the specialist

ur/ology: "science of urinary tract"; dealing with the ur/o/genit/al or ur/in/ary system and its diseases

    ur/ologist — the specialist

onc/ology: "science of tumors"; dealing with the study and treatment of tumors

    onc/ologist — the specialist

APPLICATION OF ELEMENTS
TO SOME MEDICAL CLASSIFICATIONS

Topographic Systems

Note: top/o/graph/ic: "pertaining to description of place"; system "a placing together"

body as a whole: includes the mind (psyche) and other regions which are a particular system exclusively

cardi/o/vas/cul/ar: "pertaining to the heart and vessels"; the heart and the blood vessels

digestive: the alimentary tract or canal; the tube beginning at the mouth and ending at the anus through which food is ingested, digested, and eliminated; includes the teeth, tongue, salivary glands, liver, and pancreas

end/o/crine: "secreting within"; the system of ductless glands including the thyroid, parathyroid, thymus, pituitary, pineal, adrenals

hem/ic and lymphat/ic: "pertaining to the blood and lymph"; the blood, lymph, spleen

in/tegument/ary: "pertaining to the covering (skin)"; the skin (including mucous membranes, glands of the skin, hair, nails, breast)

muscul/o/skelet/al: "pertaining to the muscles and bony framework"; the bones, muscles, joints, cartilages, bursas, ligaments, tendons

nerv/ous: the nerves including the brain and spinal cord

organs of special sense: principally sight and hearing (eyes and ears)

re/spirat/ory: "pertaining to breathing"; the nose, sinuses, larynx (voice box), trachea (windpipe), bronchial structures, lung, lung covering and chest cavity lining (pleura)

Top/o/graph/ic systems: are groupings of interconnected or interdependent organs which together accomplish some specific function. These systems form the major categories within which diseases and operations are classified for record keeping and other display and reference usage.

ur/o/genit/al: "pertaining to the urinary and genital"; kidney, bladder, urethra, internal and external reproductive organs, female genital organs during pregnancy including the fetus and fetal structures

MEDICAL TERMS USED IN THE DESCRIPTION OF DISEASES

a/chlor/hydr/ia   see chlor/hydr/ia

a/chyl/ia   (a- not + chyl- gastric juice)   "not gastric juice"; partial or complete loss of gastric juice

a/gen/e/sis   (a- not + genesis- development)   "not developed"; faulty or incomplete development

a/nom/aly   (a- not + nomaly- distributed)   "not distributed"; not in a normal or expected position

a/plas/ia   (a- not + plasia- formation, development)   "not formed"; the incomplete or faulty formation of an organ or part

a/spir/ation   (a- from ad- to + spiration- breathing)   "to breathe"; the act of breathing or drawing in; also the removal of fluids or gases from a cavity by suction

a/tres/ia   (a- not + tres- hole or opening)   "not opening"; absence or closure of a natural passage of the body

a/troph/y   (a- not + trophy- nourishment)   "not nourished"; a wasting away or decrease in size as from disuse, old age, injury or disease

abs/cess   (ab- from abs- away + cess- go)   Literally "to go away"; a localized collection of pus surrounded by inflamed tissue

ad/hes/ion   (ad- to + hesion- a sticking)   "sticking to"; the abnormal union of surfaces normally separated by the formation of new fibrous tissue; also the union of the edges of a wound

aden/o/carcin/oma   (aden- gland + carcin- cancer + oma- tumor)   "cancerous gland tumor"; a cancerous (malignant) tumor originating in glandular tissues such as the breast

aden/o/lymph/oma   (aden- gland + lymph + oma- tumor)   "tumor of the lymph gland"; an adenoma (benign tumor of gland-like structure) of a lymph organ

aden/o/my/oma   (aden- gland + my- muscle + oma- tumor)   "tumor of gland and muscle"; a benign tumor composed of muscular and glandular elements

aden/o/my/osis   (aden- gland + my- muscle + osis- condition)   "condition of muscle and gland"; the presence of endometrial (lining of the uterus) material in the myometrium (muscular layer of the wall of the uterus); also called internal endometriosis

aden/oma   (aden- gland + oma- tumor)   "tumor of gland"; a benign tumor of a gland-like structure

aero/phag/ia   (aer- air + phag- eat, swallow)   "air swallowing"; the swallowing of air expecially in hysteria

ag/glut/in/ation   (ag- from ad- to + glut- glue)   "stick to"; the process of union in the healing of a wound; also, a reaction in which particles such as red blood cells, bacteria, and virus particles tend to cluster together when suspended in a liquid

amel/o/blast/oma   (amel- enamel + blast- bud + oma- tumor)   "tumor of enamel buds or germ cells"; a tumor of the jaw formed from remnants of tooth enamel germ (bud or sprout) cells

amyl/oid   (amyl- starch + oid- resembling)   "resembling starch, starchlike"; a starchlike substance; starchy food

MEDICAL TERMS USED IN THE DESCRIPTION OF DISEASES

an/orex/ia
(an- not, lacking + orexia- desire, appetite) "lacking appetite"; pathological loss of appetite from psychic causes frequently resulting from starvation diets

ana/plast/ic
(ana- back again + plast- to form) "form back again"; characterized by reversed development

angul/ation
(angul- angle) "process or connected with an angle"; an abnormal bend or curve in an organ

bi/furc/ation
(bi- two + furc- fork) "two-forked"; branching into two parts; division into two branches

bulim/ia
(bul- cattle + lim- hunger) "literally, hungry as cattle"; an abnormal and constant craving for food

calcar/eous
(calcar- of lime) "full of lime"; containing calcium or any calcium compound

calc/ul/us
(calc- stone + ul- small) "a small stone"; solid stonelike matter composed mostly of mineral salts, found mainly in hollow organs, ducts, passages, and cysts

carcin/oma
(carcin- cancer + oma- tumor) "cancerous tumor"; a malignant tumor

cardi/algia
(cardi- heart + algia- pain) "heart pain"; heartburn; pain in the heart

caud/al/ly
(caud- tail) "toward the tail"; in a direction more toward the tail or the rear hind part of the trunk

chlor/hydr/ia
(chlor- chlorine + hydr- water) a combination meaning "hydrochloric acid" or, more specifically, "hydrochloric acid in the gastric juice," essential in breaking food down into simpler chemical compounds which can be absorbed and used by the body

a/chlorhydria
(a- not + chlorhydria) "not hydrochloric acid"; absence of hydrochloric acid from the gastric juice

hyper/chlorhydria
(hyper- above, excessive + chlorhydria) "excessive hydrochloric acid"; the presence of a greater than typical proportion of hydrochloric acid in the gastric juice, especially characteristic of various pathological states such as ulceration

hypo/chlorhydria
(hypo- below, deficient + chlorhydria) "deficient hydrochloric acid"; deficiency of hydrochloric acid in the gastric juice

chol/angi/oma
(chole- bile + angi- vessel, duct + oma- tumor) "tumor of bile duct"; a tumor of the bile ducts

chondr/oma
(chondr- cartilage + oma- tumor) "tumor of cartilage"; a tumor composed of cartilage tissue

con/cret/ion
(con- together + cret- grow) "grow together"; a hard mass formed in a body cavity or in tissue

con/stip/ation
(con- together + stip- press) "press together"; abnormally delayed or infrequent movement of dry hardened feces

con/tract/ure
(con- together + tract- draw) "draw together"; deformity or distortion produced by scar tissue or a permanent shortening of muscles, tendons, or fascia

MEDICAL TERMS USED IN THE DESCRIPTION OF DISEASES

cyst

(cyst- pouch, bladder) "pouch"; a pouch lacking an opening but having a membrane and developing in a natural cavity of the body, in the substance of an organ, or in an abnormal structure such as a tumor; also a bladder, especially applied to the urinary and gall bladders

di/lat/ation

(di- from dis- apart + lat- wide) "wide apart"; the condition of being stretched beyond normal dimensions especially as a result of overwork or disease

di/vert/ic/ul/ation

(di from de- away from + vert- turn) "a turning away from"; the formation of abnormal pouches or sacs opening from a hollow organ such as the intestine or bladder

dia/rrhea

(dia- through + rrhe- flow) "flow through"; an abnormal frequency of discharge of more or less fluid waste products from the bowels

dis/loc/ation

(dis- apart + loc- place) "apart from place"; displacement of one or more bones at a joint; compare displacement, ectopia

dis/place/ment

(dis- apart + place-) "apart from place"; ectopia (out of place); removal from normal position or place; generally applied to other than out-of-position bones (dislocation) such as mental substitutes for reality, an out-of-place condition of the stomach, tissue change of position as a result of the pressure; compare dislocation, ectopia

dis/tort/ion

(dis- apart + tort- twist) "twisting apart"; the state of being twisted out of a natural or normal state or position

dors/al/ly

(dors- back) "backwardly"; in a back position or direction

duplic/ation

(duplic- double, twofold) "doubling"; the action or process of doubling especially applied to abnormal doublings or duplications in fetal development

dys/phag/ia

(dys- bad, difficult + phag- swallowing) "difficult swallowing"; difficulty in swallowing due to disease or accident

dys/plas/ia

(dys- bad, abnormal + plasia- development, growth) "abnormal development"; abnormal growth or development as of organs, tissues or cells

ef/fer/ent

(ef- from, ex- from, away from + fer- carry) "carry away from"; bearing or conducting outward from a part or organ; specifically, the conveying of nervous impulses from a center

e/long/ation

(e- from ex- from, away from + long- far, distant) "far away from"; the process or condition of increasing in length

e/ruct/ation

(e- from ex- from, forth + ruct- belch) "belch forth"; the act of belching gas from the stomach

ec/top/ia

(e from ex- from, away from + top- place) "away from place"; an abnormal congenital or acquired position of an organ or part such as the heart, crystalline lens, testicle, bladder; compare dislocation, displacement

em/bol/ism

(em- from in- in + bol- throw) "thrown in, stopped'; the sudden blocking of an artery by a clot or obstruction carried by the blood stream

em/bol/us

(em- from in- in + bol- throw) "throw in, stopper"; the clot or plug obstructing the blood flow in a blood vessel

MEDICAL TERMS USED IN THE DESCRIPTION OF DISEASES

end/arter/itis   (end- within + arter- artery + itis- inflammation) "inflammation within artery"; inflammation of the innermost lining of an artery

epi/derm/oid   (epi- above + derm- skin + oid- resembling) "resembling upper skin"; resembling the top skin layer (epidermis); composed of elements like those of the epidermis

epi/gastr/ium   (epi- above, over + gastr- stomach) "over the stomach"; the upper middle region of the abdomen

ex/trus/ion   (ex- from, out + trus- push, thrust) "push out"; a forcing out or expulsion; the condition of a tooth which extends above the bite line of the surrounding teeth

extra/vas/ation   (extra- outside, beyond + vas- vessel) "outside a vessel"; discharge or escape, as of blood into the tissues

fibr/o/sarc/oma   (fibr- fiber + sarc- flesh + oma- tumor) "tumor of fiber and flesh"; a tumor composed of fleshy and fibrous elements

fibr/oma   (fibr- fiber + oma- tumor) "fibrous tumor"; a tumor composed mainly of fibrous elements

fibr/osis   (fibr- fiber + osis- condition) "fibrous condition"; the formation of fibrous tissue; the degeneration of fibrous structures

fist/ul/a   (fistul- pipe) "pipe or passage"; an abnormal passage from an abscess, cavity, or hollow organ to the skin or to another abscess, cavity, or hollow organ

flacc/id   (flacc- flabby) "flabby"; weak, soft, lax; lacking tone, resilience, or firmness, especially muscles

fus/ion   (fus- melt) "union as if by melting"; the abnormal coherence of adjacent parts or bodies

gangli/o/neur/oma   (gangli- knot, swelling + neur- nerv + oma- tumor) "knotty nerve tumor"; a tumor growing from a nerve cell composed mainly of ganglion material; a tumor consisting of nerve and ganglion tissues

gangren/e   (gangren- gnawing away, an eating sore) "an eating away"; death of tissue, usually resulting from loss of blood supply

gli/osis   (gli- glue + osis- condition) "gluelike condition"; disease associated with excessive development of the supporting structure of nerve tissue

gran/ul/o/cyt/ic   (granul- little grain + cyt- cell) "pertaining to cells of small grainlike construction"; pertaining to a cell composed of grainlike particles

gran/ul/oma   (granul- little grain, little particle + oma- tumor) "grainy tumor"; a tumor or neoplasm made up of grainlike (granulation) tissue; a mass of chronically inflamed tissue marked by the formation of granulations

halit/osis   (halit- breath + osis- condition) "breath condition"; bad breath; offensive breath

hem/angi/oma   (hem- blood + angi- vessel + oma- tumor) "blood vessel tumor"; a usually benign tumor made up of blood vessels

hem/o/glob/in   (hem- blood + glob from globul- tiny ball) "tiny blood ball"; the red coloring matter of the red blood corpuscles serving to carry oxygen from the lungs to the tissues and carbon dioxide from the tissues to the lungs

MEDICAL TERMS USED IN THE DESCRIPTION OF DISEASES

hepat/o/megal/y   (hepat- liver + megaly- enlarged) "enlarged liver"; enlargement of the liver

hern/ia   (hern- intestine, entrails) "entrails condition"; rupture; the protrusion of all or part of an organ through a tear in the wall of the surrounding structure, especially the protrusion of the intestine through the abdominal muscles

hydr/o/peri/ton/eum   (hydr- water, fluid + peri- around + ton- stretch, stretched) "fluid in the stretched around"; note the peritoneum is the membrane which lines (stretched around) the abdominal cavity; ascites; abnormal accumulation of fluid in the abdominal cavity

hyper/chlor/hydr/ia   see chlorhydria

hyper/motil/ity   (hyper- above, excessive + motil- movement) "excessive movement"; abnormal or excessive movement; specifically, movement (motility) of all or part of the gastrointestinal tract; compare hypomotility

hyper/plas/ia   (hyper- above, excessive + plasia- formation) "excessive formation"; an abnormal or unusual increase in the elements composing a part such as the cells of a tissue

hyper/secret/ion   (hyper- above, excessive + secret- set apart) "excessive setting apart or separation"; excessive segregating or releasing of some material to perform a function (salivation) or for excretion (urination)

hyper/troph/y   (hyper- above, more than normal + trophy- nourishment, growth) "more than normal growth"; a considerable increase in the size of an organ or tissue

hypo/chlor/hydr/ia   see chlorhydria

hyper/motil/ity   (hyper- above, excessive + motil- movement) "excessive movement"; abnormal or excessive movement; specifically, movement (motility) of all or part of the gastrointestinal tract; compare hypomotility

im/pact/ion   (im- from, in- within, together + pact- press) "press together"; the condition of being firmly lodged (packed); specifically, of teeth which are so imbedded as to prevent eruption, or hardened feces in the rectum

in/carcer/ation   (in- in, within + carcer- prison) "imprisonment"; constricted, abnormal retention or confinement of a body part; specifically the constriction of the neck of a hernial sac

in/clus/ion   (in- in + clus- close) "closed or shut in"; anything that is enclosed; specifically, a lifeless constituent of a cell, or a tooth so surrounded with bony material that it is unable to erupt

in/continence   (in- not, lack + contin- hold, contain) "not holding"; lacking control; unrestrained; especially, uncontrolled sexual desire or inability to contain a bodily discharge such as urine

in/volut/ion   (in- in, inner + volut- rolling) "an inner rolling or rolling within"; a shrinking such as the return of the uterus to its former size after delivery, or the shriveling of an organ in an aged person, or the decrease in bodily vigor in women during menopause

leio/my/o/sarc/oma   (leio- smooth + my- muscle + sarc- flesh + oma- tumor) "smooth, muscle, fleshy tumor"; a fleshy tumor containing smooth muscle elements

MEDICAL TERMS USED IN THE DESCRIPTION OF DISEASES

les/ion
(les- injure, hurt) "an injury"; injury; impairment; flaw; an abnormal change or loss of function in a part or organ due to injury or disease

lig/ation
(lig- tie, bind) "tied or bound"; something that binds; also the surgical act of binding or tieing

lip/o/sarc/oma
(lip- fat + sarc- flesh + oma- tumor) "fat, fleshy tumor", a fleshy tumor containing fatty elements

lip/oma
(lip- fat + oma- tumor) "fatty tumor"; a tumor made up of fat cells

lymph/angi/oma
(lymph- watery fluid, lymph + angi- vessel + oma- tumor) "lymph vessel tumor"; a tumor formed of lymphatic vessels

lymph/o/sarc/oma
(lymph- watery fluid, lymph + sarc- flesh + oma- tumor) "lymph, fleshy tumor"; a general term applied to malignant neoplastic disorders of lympoid tissue, particularly a malignant tumor which spreads (metastisizes) to adjacent glands

lymph/oid
(lymph- watery fluid, lymph + oid- resembling) "resembling lymph, lymphlike"; resembling the tissue characteristics of lymph glands

malign/ancy
(mal- bad, evil, or malign- acting evilly) "bad action, evil action", a cancerous tumor; exhibiting cancerous qualities

medull/ary
(medull- marrow, pith) "of the pith or inner substance"; resembling marrow; pertaining to the innermost part (pith) of an organ or structure

melan/oma
(melan- black + oma- tumor) "black tumor"; a tumor made up of black-pigmented cells

melan/osis
(melan- black + osis- condition) "black condition"; a condition characterized by deposits of black or other pigmentary deposits in the tissues of the body

mes/o/thel/i/oma
(mes- middle + thel- nipple, cellular tissue + oma- tumor) "middle cellular tissue tumor"; a tumor derived from tissue such as that lining the peritoneum or pleura (mesothelial)

meta/bol/ism
(meta- beyond, change + bol- throw, thrust) "thrust beyond"; the chemical and physical processes (changes) continuously going on in the body and its constituent parts; the bodily processes of assmiliating food and breaking food down into simpler substances to provide repairs and energy

meta/sta/tic
(meta- beyond, change + sta- stand, place) "pertaining to placing beyond, spreading"; pertaining to the spread of disease from one part of the body to another

my/o/blast/oma
(my- muscle + blast- bud, sprout + oma- tumor) "muscle bud tumor"; a tumor in the muscle made up of groups of cells which resemble primitive (sprout) muscle cells

myel/oma
(myel- marrow, spinal cord + oma- tumor) "bone marrow tumor"; a tumor of the bone marrow

necr/osis
(necr- dead + osis- condition) "dead condition"; death of living tissue as may be caused by loss of blood supply, burning, local lesion of a disease, or injury

neo/plas/m
(neo- new + plas- growth) "a new growth"; any new or abnormal growth such as a tumor; may be benign, potentially malignant, or malignant

MEDICAL TERMS USED IN THE DESCRIPTION OF DISEASES

neur/o/fibr/oma (neur- nerv + fibr- fiber + oma- tumor) "nerve and fiber tumor"; a fibrous tumor originating in the fibrous tissue of a nerve sheath

non/fus/ion (non- not, lack + fus- melt, join) "lack of joining"; failure of parts, such as the edges of a wound, to properly join

ob/stip/ation (ob- completely, totally + stip- press) "pressing completely or totally"; severe and persistent constipation

oc/clus/ion (oc- from ob- completely, totally + clus- close) "close completely"; shutting off or obstruction of something such as the obstruction of the flow of blood to the heart (coronary occlusion); a closing or shutting such as the meeting of the teeth when the jaws are closed

opac/ity (opac- dark, shaded) "condition of darkness"; darkness; a dark (opaque) spot on a normally transparent structure such as the cornea or lens of the eye

oste/oma (oste- bone + oma- tumor) "bone tumor"; a tumor composed of bone tissue

papill/ary (papill- nipple) "nipple-like"; pertaining to a nipple or resembling a nipple such as the small protrubances on the upper surface of the tongue

papill/oma (papill- nipple + oma- tumor) "nipple-like tumor"; a benign tumor such as a wart or pimple growing on the surface of the skin (epithelium)

par/en/chym/atous (par from para- beside, alongside + en from in- in + chym from chein- to pour) "relating to pour in beside (from the belief that the tissue of internal organs was poured in by the blood vessels)"; the essential elements of an organ (as a gland) or an abnormal growth (as a tumor) as distinguished from its supporting framework

par/esis (par- from para- beside, at the side + esis- let go, send) "action of letting go, letting fall at the side"; slight or partial paralysis

para/sym/path/etic (para- beyond, beside + sym- with + path- feeling) "feeling with beside or beyond"; properly the parasympathetic nervous system; the part of the nervous system whose functions include the constriction of the pupils of the eyes, the slowing of the heartbeat, and the stimulation of certain digestive glands

path/ogen/ic (path- feeling, suffering, disease + gen- producing, originating) "production of suffering or disease"; pertaining to the production or development of disease

peri/ton/eal (peri- around, surrounding + ton- stretch) "stretched around"; pertaining to the membrane lining the abdominal cavity

petechiae (petechiae- small spots produced in some infectious diseases) "contagious disease spot"; small, pinpoint, nonraised, perfectly round, purplish red spots appearing on the skin in some contagious diseases such as typhoid fever spots

pica (pica- magpie, a bird that eats everything) "as non-discriminating as a magpie"; a craving for unnatural articles of food brought on by nutritional deficiencies or occurring in insanity; also, sometimes exhibited during pregnancy

MEDICAL TERMS USED IN THE DESCRIPTION OF DISEASES

plasm/a   (plasm- something formed) "formation"; the fluid part of the blood, lymph, milk, or intramuscular liquid, especially the fluid part of the blood (as distinguished from the corpuscles) used for transfusions

plate/let/s   (plate- from platy- broad, flat + let- little) "little plates"; a tiny flattened body, especially any of the small disks containing no hemoglobin found in the blood and associated with the process of blood clotting

poly/dips/ia   (poly- many, much + dips- thirst) "much thirst"; excessive or abnormal thirst

poly/p   (poly- many + p shortened from pous- from pod- foot) "many feet"; a protruding growth from any mucous membrane, especially the mucous membrane of the nose. (the "many feet" applies to the roots of the growth)

pre/malign/ant   (pre- before + malign- cancerous) "before malignancy"; preceeding the development of malignancy; precancerous

pro/lap/se   (pro- before, forward + lapse- falling) "falling forward"; the falling or slipping out of place of an internal organ

pro/trus/ion   (pro- before, forth + trusion- thrusting) "thrusting forth"; a thrusting or jutting out

proct/algia   (proct- rectum + algia- pain) "pain in the rectum"; pain in the rectum

prol/i/fer/ation   (prol- offspring + fer- bear, carry) "bearing offspring"; multiply rapidly; the reproduction or multiplication of similar forms, especially of cells and morbid cysts

pt/osis   (pt- fall + osis- condition) "falling condition"; a prolapse; the falling of some organ or part, especially the drooping of the upper eyelid, caused by the paralysis of its muscle

ptyal/ism   (ptyal- saliva) "action pertaining to spit"; excessive secretion of saliva

pyl/or/ic   (pylor- gatekeeper) "pertaining to gatekeeping"; pertaining to the opening (gate) from the stomach into the first part of the small intestine (the pylorus)

rupt/ure   (rupt- break) "act of breaking"; breaking apart; bursting; a forcible tearing or bursting of an organ or part, as of a blood vessel, the bladder, etc.

scirrh/ous   (scirrh- hard) "resembling hardness"; resembling a hard cancerous tumor

scler/osis   (scler- hard + osis- condition) "hard condition"; a pathological hardening of tissue as in arteriosclerosis, multiple sclerosis

sen/ile   (sen- old) "having to do with age"; typical of or resulting from old age, especially the mental impairment characterized by confusion, memory loss, etc.

sin/us   (sin- curve, fold) "a fold"; any of various cavities, hollows and passages, especially the air cavities in the skull opening into the nasal passages

squam/ous   (squam- scale) "scalelike"; like, formed of, or covered with scales

sta/sis   (sta- stand) "condition of standing or stoppage"; a stoppage of the flow of some fluid in the body such as blood; reduced peristalsis of the intestines resulting in the retention of feces

MEDICAL TERMS USED IN THE DESCRIPTION OF DISEASES

strangul/ation (strangul- a squeezing, choking) "a squeezing or constriction"; inordinate constriction or compression of a tube or a part (as the throat or bowel), especially to a degree that causes a suspension of breathing, circulation, or passage of contents

strict/ure (strict- compress, draw tight) "compression"; an abnormal narrowing of a passage in the body; stenosis

sym/path/etic (sym from syn- with + path- disease, feeling) "pertaining to feeling with"; the sympathetic nerve or system of nerves

sym/path/ic/o/blast/oma (sym from syn- with + path- feeling, disease + blast- bud + oma- tumor) or (sympathic- pertaining to the sympathetic nerves + blast- bud, sprout + oma- tumor) "sympathetic cell bud tumor"; a malignant tumor composed of primitive cells which develop into a sympathetic nerve cell

terat/oma (terat- monster + oma- tumor) "monstrous tumor"; a tumor containing various kinds of embryonic tissue as of hair, teeth, bone, muscle, cartilage

thromb/o/cyt/e (thromb- clot + cyt- cell) "clotting cell"; a small blood cell that initiates the process of blood clotting; platelet

thromb/osis (thromb- clot + osis- condition) "clotting condition"; coagulation (clotting) of the blood in the heart or a blood vessel forming a clot

thromb/us (thromb- clot) "a clot"; the clot attached at the site of the thrombosis

tors/ion (tors- twist) "a twisting"; the act of turning or twisting; the state of being twisted; the twisting of a body part on its own axis such as a loop of intestine; or the condition of a tooth when it is turned on its long axis

troph/ic (troph- nourishment, growth) "pertaining to nourishment"; of nutrition; having to do with the processes of nutrition

tum/or (tum- swell) "a swelling"; a swelling on some part of the body, especially a mass of new tissue growth; neoplasm

tympan/ite/s (tympan- a drum) "drumlike"; a distension of the abdomen by the accumulation of gas or air in the intestines or abdominal cavity. "Tight as a drum"

xer/o/stom/ia (xer- dry + stom- mouth) "dry mouth condition"; abnormal dryness of the mouth due to insufficient secretions

CLASSIFICATION OF OPERATIVE PROCEDURES

PURPOSE OF THIS SECTION

Many of the elements discussed in Medical Terminology are directly concerned with operative procedures. Operative procedures are descriptions of the therapeutic measures which physicians perform for the alleviation or cure of disease and injury. In this section we will discuss the elements used in operative procedures. This discussion will serve to broaden your knowledge of the application of elements as they relate to operations and give you a better appreciation of the meanings of elements as they relate to and differ from each other.

Organization of Operative Procedures

Within body systems and the major organs which are parts of that body system, operative procedures are classified under the following major categories:

INCISION

EXCISION

AMPUTATION

INTRODUCTION

ENDOSCOPY

REPAIR

DESTRUCTION

SUTURE

MANIPULATION

INCISION **in/cis/ion:** a "cutting into"; a cut made into a tissue or organ

Kinds of incisions:
-/o/tom/y: a "cutting"; the general word ending used to indicate a cutting into a tissue or organ; section

-cent/esis: a "pricking"; surgical puncture; a needling

tran/sect/ion: a "cutting across"; a "cross cut"; a long cut; a division by cutting into sections

EXCISION **ex/cis/ion:** a "cutting out"; surgical removal

Kinds of excision:

-ec/tom/y: "cutting out"; the general word ending used to indicate surgical removal

CLASSIFICATION OF
OPERATIVE PROCEDURES

ex/cis/ion of les/ion (local ex/cis/ion of les/ion) surgical removal in which the tissue to be removed (ex/cis/ed) lies within a relatively narrow area; contrast with re/sect/ion

A les/ion (les- means to hurt or to injure: an injury or other change in an organ resulting in impairment or loss of function.) Tumors, cysts, ulcers are examples of les/ion/s

Loc/al (pertaining to place) denotes a particular part or specific area of the body; not general; not extensive

re/sect/ion: "cut back"; ex/cis/ion of a considerable portion of an organ or structure; sometimes used to indicate an excision over a wider or deeper area than is implied in a generalized -ec/tom/y or "excision of lesion"

radic/al ex/cis/ion: "root cutting out"; going to the "root" or source of a les/ion or other cause; similar to our expression "root out" by which we mean complete removal or eradication

bi/ops/y: "seeing life"; "viewing life"; the ex/cis/ion of a bit of living tissue from the body for diagnostic examination

AMPUTATION from am- (amphi-) "two ways" plus -put/ate "clean, trim, prune"; the surgical cutting off (an arm, leg, etc.)

dis/articul/ation: (articul- means "joint"; same as arthr-); "joint apart"; the act of surgically disjointing; separation at the joint

INTRODUCTION intro/duct/ion: the act of "leading into"; a putting in; insertion

Essentially, intro/duct/ion indicates the insertion or putting of something into the body

in/ject/ion: (ject- means "throw"; a tra/ject/ory is the course followed by something thrown; to e/ject is to throw out); "throw or force in"; the act of forcing or driving (usually a fluid) into some part of the body

trans/fus/ion: (fus- means "pour", "melt"; to re/fuse is to pour back; give back; put back) "pour across"; the act of pouring across or transferring; specifically, to transfer (blood, blood plasma, saline solution, etc.) into a blood vessel, usually a vein

im/plant/ation: "plant into"; insertion of a substance, organ, or piece of living tissue into the body

in/sert/ion: the act of putting or setting something into something else; the act of putting something (usually a device) into the body.

The "something" (devices) may be wires, pins, nails; dentures or other prosthetic devices; orthodontic appliances, pacemakers, etc.

Or, the device may be briefly introduced such as in:

cath/et/er/ization — the insertion of a cath/et/er for the introduction or withdrawal of fluids

in/tub/ation — the insertion of a tube, usually for the passage of air or fluids

CLASSIFICATION OF
OPERATIVE PROCEDURES

ENDOSCOPY *endo/scop/y* "observe within"; the act of examining visually the inside of a hollow organ of the body

> The instrument used for such examination is an endo/scop/e. Endo/scop/es have developed into versatile devices. They are not limited to viewing alone but may also be equipped to obtain biopsies, excise tissue, drain fluids, remove foreign bodies, divide adhesions, insert and inject substances

REPAIR to put back in good condition after damage; to restore; renew; set right; remedy

> **-plasty** is the word ending used to generally indicate repair

> **plast/ic repair of. . .** is also used in the same sense of -plasty ore repair

The element plas- means "to form"; "to mold". We have learned that the word ending -plas/ia means "forming", "growth", "development". Plast/ic surgery is the branch of surgery concerned with the repair or restoration of lost, injured, or deformed parts of the body, chiefly by the transfer of tissue. Plasma (sometimes shortened to plasm) means "something formed"; used mostly to indicate the fluid portions of the blood

Plast/ic repair or -plasty can encompass such surgical procedures on body parts as:

> LENGTHENING
>
> SHORTENING
>
> RESTORATION
>
> RECONSTRUCTION
>
> REVISION

Other repairs are designated as:
> **graft** transplantation of a piece of skin, bone, or other living tissue from one body, or place on a body, to another

>> **-stom/y** — "making a mouth"; a surgical opening into a specified part or organ frequently for drainage

>>> **-ana/stomy (ana/stom/osis)** — "make a mouth again"; interconnection; surgical joining of one hollow or tubular organ with another

> **fistul/ization:** the surgical creation of an opening into a hollow organ, or of an opening between two structures which were not previously connected

> **open reduction:** (a re/duct/ion "lead back" is the correction of a fracture or hernia): correction (re/duct/ion) of a fracture after exposing the fracture by an incision

> **-pexy:** word ending meaning fastening, fixing in place; securing; making fast fixation: the operation of holding, suturing, or fastening in a fixed position
> suspension: — "hang up"; to hang from a support

CLASSIFICATION OF
OPERATIVE PROCEDURES

-desis: word ending meaning joining or tieing

    fus/ion — to bind together; frequently the immobilizing of a joint; arthr/o/desis; artificial ankyl/o/sis. (Ankylosis means a "sticking together" condition, artificial ankylosis means a surgical "sticking together" or fus/ion of a joint, hence, is synonymous with arthr/o/desis.)

    stabilization — to make steady or firm; again, frequently by fusing some of the bones in the joint; arthr/o/desis

    trans/plant/ation: "planting across"; to transfer (tissue or an organ) from one individual, or part of the body, to another; graft

DESTRUCTION   the act of obliterating, doing away with de/bride/ment (literally to unbridle); the cutting away of dead or contaminated tissue from a wound to prevent infection

    -clas/is: "breaking"; the act of breaking

        fracturing — the surgical breaking of a bone to correct a deformity

        re/fracturing — the operation of breaking over again a bone which has been fractured and has united with a deformity

    -tripsy, -trity: word endings indicating the act of crushing

        crushing — applying pressure so as to destroy a structure or substances such as stones (calculi) in the body

    -lysis: word ending indicating loosening, freeing, or division of adhesions (adhesions denote the fibrous tissues which join together body parts which normally are separate; it typically results from inflammation): the removal of adhesions; the surgical severing of the fibers which are abnormally uniting body parts

        Note: "adhesion" carries the same "sticking together" idea that we use in the word "adhesive"

    stripping: An operative procedure for varicose veins in which large sections of the veins are removed

SUTURE: the act or method of joining together the two edges of a wound or incision by stitching or similar means

    -rrhaphy: word ending denoting suturing

Suturing may be applied in:

    closure of wound
    closure of fistula

    resuturing, that is, stitching a wound again if the first suturing fails to hold

    lig/ation, that is, tying off blood vessels or other structures during the performance of an operation

CLASSIFICATION OF
OPERATIVE PROCEDURES

MANIPULATION   (literally, to operate with the hand or hands) treatment by using the hands

You may be familiar with some conditions which are treated by the skillful manipulation of the physician's hands:

In deliveries at term:

obstetric delivery

conversion of position   in case the fetus needs to be turned in the uterus (breech presentation)

obstetric extraction   in the event the mother needs assistance in expelling the fetus from the uterus

version, a term to cover a variety of internal and external manipulations to ease or expedite delivery. (remember vers- "turn"?)

application of or delivery by forceps,   the use of a tong-like instrument (forceps) designed to extract the fetus by the head from the birth canal

In dislocations and simple fractures:

manipulation and application of   plaster, splint, or traction apparatus

closed reduction of fractures, that is, fractures which can be corrected with manipulation without the need for incision to expose the fracture

Removal of   drains, dressings, packing, sutures, wires, etc.

Dilation or stretching

-tasia, tasis: word endings denoting the act of enlarging a passage or hollow organ by stretching

ALPHABETICAL LIST OF ELEMENTS

ELEMENT	LESSON	ELEMENT	LESSON	ELEMENT	LESSON	ELEMENT	LESSON
ab	11	dynam	10	mani	3	proli	11
acousti	6	dys	9	mast	3	proxim	II-2
acro	3	ectasis	4	maxill	10	pseud	II-1
aden	1	ectomy	1	mechano	10	psycho	2
adnexa	7	edema	8	med	II-2	ptosis	3
adreno	12	emesis	4	megal	1	ptyal	8
aer	8	en	9	melan	4	puer	11
algia	2	encephal	6	mening	5	pulmon	8
alveol	8	end	2	ment	7	pyle, pyloro	5
ambi	II-1	enter	1	meta	II-2	rachi	9
ameb	10	ependym	8	metabole	8	radi	8
amphi	II-1	epi	3	metr	10	radic	8
an, a	10	erythro	4	mi	II-2	ramus	10
angi	1	esophag	12	micr	9	ren	6
ante	11	esthesia	4	morph	II-2	retro	3
anti	5	eu	II-1	my	2	rhin	1
antr	7	eury	II-2	myco	5	rhexis	3
apo	II-2	ex	11	myel	5	rrhag	II-2
appendic	12	fac	II-2	myring	4	rrhaphy	3
arter	12	fascia	7	necr	II-2	rrhe	II-2
arthr	1	fiss	II-1	neo	10	rug	6
asthenia	7	fistul	8	nephr	1	sacro	12
astr	7	furca	8	neuro	10	salpingo	6
aur	6	gangli	9	ocul	7	sarc	11
auto	3	gastr	1	odont	4	schiz	II-1
basi	12	gemin	9	oid	2	scirr	7
benign	4	gen	3	olfact	II-1	sclera	7
bi	12	ger	II-1	ologist	1	scol	II-2
bili	5	gingiv	1	ology	1	scope	2
blast	II-2	glom	11	oma	1	sedat	8
blephar	1	glosso	3	oment	8	semen	4
brachy	II-1	glyco	8	onco	5	semi	10
brady	4	grad	9	onych	5	sept	7
bronch	12	gram	3	oophor	8	sinus	7
bucco	6	gran	9	ophthalm, opt	2	somato	7
burso	3	gravid	8	or	5	somni	11
calc	9	gyn	II-1	orth	II-1	spas	11
cantho	4	hallux	5	orchi	6	spasm	1
capit	II-1	helio	7	osis	1	sphenic	5
carcin	3	hem(at)	2	osmo	10	spiro	5
cardi	1	hemi	2	ost	2	splanchn	II-2
cata	II-1	hepat	1	ostomy	2	splen	12
cau	II-1	heter	II-1	oto	5	spondyl	4
cauda	4	histo	6	otomy	1	squam	5
cec	5	hom	II-1	ovar	5	sta	II-2
cele	4	hormone	10	ovario	12	steno	4
celio	4	hydro	3	pachy	II-1	stoma	6
centesis	5	hyper	2	palpebr	6	strept	3
cephal	3	hypno	7	pan	10	strict	10
cerebr	1	hypo	2	para	2	sub	5
cervic	2	hyster	2	pariet	8	supra	3
cheil	4	iasis	4	part	7	syn, sym	10
cheir, chir	9	ile	12	path	1	tarso	7
chole	2	ili	12	pect	II-2	tarso	9
chondr	2	infer	II-1	pelvis	12	tegument	10
cilia	6	infra	11	penia	3	tens	11
cine	9	inter	11	peps, pept	9	thalam	6
clas	II-1	intra	11	per	II-2	thel	11
col	12	iris	8	peri	9	therap	12
colla	9	iso	7	pexy	5	therm	10
colpo	6	itis	1	phage	8	thorac	5
contra	4	kerat	8	phak	10	thromb	11
cor	6	labi	9	pharmac	11	thyro	12
corne	8	lacrim	5	pharyng	12	ton	II-2
cost	3	lact	5	phleb	6	tope	7
crani	2	lal	11	phob	9	trachel	7
crine	7	lapar	7	phon	6	trans	4
cryo	11	laryng	12	phot	9	traumat	10
cut	9	later	9	phrag	II-1	tri	12
cyan	2	leio	6	phren	8	trich	10
cyst	2	lept	II-2	physio	6	trip	3
cyt	4	leuk	4	pilo	6	trophy	3
dacry	7	lien	11	plak	8	tumor	11
dactyl	8	lig	12	plasia	6	turbin	10
dendr	6	lingua	4	plast	1	tympan	6
dent	3	lip	2	platy	II-1	ureter	12
dermat	1	lith	2	plegia	11	utero	12
desis	3	lobo	4	pleur	9	umbilic	6
di	II-2	lumbo	11	plexus	6	vaso	4
dia	II-2	lymph	II-2	pneum	8	vena	12
digit	9	lysis	2	pod	7	ventr	II-1
dis	II-2	macro	11	poly	10	vert	II-1
dors	9	macul	5	post	10	vesic	5
duct	II-1	mal	11	poster	II-1	vestibule	11
duodeno	12	malacia	1	pre	10	viscero	5
dura	7	malign	7	pro	9	volv	II-2
dyn	3	mamm	9	proct	2	vulse	10
						xer	II-2

ALPHABETICAL LIST OF ELEMENTS, AUDIONYMS (Where Applicable) AND MEANINGS

Description of Code

0 = One of the 350 elements taught in this course
1 = Word terminal from the Reading Assignment
2 = Element developed in the Reading Assignment
3 = Element which you will recognize through its use in common words or as discussed under Familiar Elements
4 = Element used in Medical Terms Used in Description of Diseases

CODE	ELEMENT	AUDIONYM	MEANING
1	a		noun ending, name of thing from a root
0	ab	Abe	away from, not
3	abdomin		the abdomen, belly
1	ac		affected by, having, one who is affected by
1	ac		comparing "pertaining to," 'affected by'
1	ac		pertaining to
0	acousti	a cue stick	hearing, sound
0	acro	acrobat	extremities
2	acro		farthest ends plus all parts leading to
2	acus, acous		sound
1	ad		toward, in the direction of
2	ad		to, toward
0	aden	a den	gland
0	adnexa	annex	ties, connections
0	adreno		adrenal gland
1	ae		plural ending for words ending in a
0	aer	air (plane)	air
1	al		pertaining to
2	alg		pain
2	algeo		pain
2	algesi		pain, sensitivity to pain
0	algia	algae	painful condition, pain
2	algio		pain
0	alveol	owl field	cavity, socket
0	ambi, ambo	amp, bee	both, around, on both sides, (ambo, amb, am, an)
0	ameb	a me	change
4	amel		enamel
4	amyl		starch
0	amphi, ampho	amp, feet	around, on both sides, in two ways
0	an, a	an A	without, not
1	an, ian		of, belonging to, person associated with
3	ana, ano		up, back, again, throughout
1	ance, ancy		state of condition, the act of
0	angi	angel	vessel, usually blood
2	angin		a choking, strangling
4	angul		angle
2	aniso		not equal, inequality
1	ant		pertaining to, having characteristics of

ALPHABETICAL LIST OF ELEMENTS, AUDIONYMS (Where Applicable) AND MEANINGS

Description of Code

0 = One of the 350 elements taught in this course
1 = Word terminal from the Reading Assignment
2 = Element developed in the Reading Assignment
3 = Element which you will recognize through its use in common words or as discussed under Familiar Elements
4 = Element used in Medical Terms Used in Description of Diseases

CODE	ELEMENT	AUDIONYM	MEANING
0	ante	ant tea	before
0	anti	ant eye	against
2	anti		counteracting, preventing, supressing
0	antr	ant tree	cavity, chamber
0	apo	apple	away from, from, separation, lack
0	appendic		appendix
1	ar		pertaining to, having a connection with
0	arter		artery
0	arthr	art	joint
1	ary		pertaining to, having a connection with
0	asthenia	his thin knee	weakness
0	astr	astronaut	star-shaped
1	ate		perform, put into action, bring about
1	ation		a process, condition, action
2	atrophy		"not growth," wasting away, decrease
0	aur	"R"	ear
0	auto	auto	self
2	auto		self caused, occurring within one's body
0	basi		base
2	basi		bottom, lowest part, foundation
0	benign	bee "9"	mild, not cancerous
2	benign		favorable for recovery
0	bi		two, double, both
0	bili	bill	bile
2	bin		two, both
3	bio, bi		life
0	blast	blast	bud, shoot, sprout, embryonic cell
0	blephar	blue fur	eyelid
6	bol		throw
0	brachy	brake	short
0	brady	braid	slow
3	brevi		short
0	bronch		bronchus
0	bucco	bucket	cheek
2	bucco		as landmark
4	bul		cattle
0	burso	purse sew	sac
0	calc	calculator	heel, stone
4	calcar		of lime

ALPHABETICAL LIST OF ELEMENTS, AUDIONYMS (Where Applicable) AND MEANINGS

Description of Code

0 = One of the 350 elements taught in this course
1 = Word terminal from the Reading Assignment
2 = Element developed in the Reading Assignment
3 = Element which you will recognize through its use in common words or as discussed under Familiar Elements
4 = Element used in Medical Terms Used in Description of Diseases

CODE	ELEMENT	AUDIONYM	MEANING
0	cantho	can throw	angle at the end of the eyelid
0	capit, cep	cap	head
4	carcer		prison
0	carcin	car sign	cancer
0	cardi	card	heart
0	cata, cath	catalog	down, lower, under, complete (also kath)
0	cau, caus	cough	burn, burning heat, cauter-searing, burning
0	cauda	cod liver oil	tail
2	cauda		"the rear end," directional use
3	cav, cavit		hollow
0	cec	seek	blind passage
0	cele	seal	hernia, tumor, or swelling
0	celio	ceiling dome	abdomen
2	celio		any large cavity of the body esp. abdomen
0	centesis	cent	puncture
0	cephal	sieve fall	head
0	cerebr	zebra	brain
0	cervic	serve hic	neck
4	cess		go
0	cheil	cow	lip
4	chein		to pour
0	cheir, chir	care (package)	hand
4	chlor		chlorine
0	chole	coal	bile
2	chole		gall
0	chondr	cone door	cartilage
4	chyl		gastric juice
0	cilia	ceiling	eyelash
2	cilia		hairlike projection
0	cine	Sen Sen	move, movement
3	circum		around, about, on all sides
0	clas, clad	class	break, destroy
1	cle		small, little
4	clus		to close
2	coel		hollow
0	col		colon
0	colla	cola	glue, gelatin-like
0	colpo	cold bow	hollow, vagina
3	com, con		with, together, completely (col, cor)

ALPHABETICAL LIST OF ELEMENTS, AUDIONYMS (Where Applicable) AND MEANINGS

Description of Code

0 = One of the 350 elements taught in this course
1 = Word terminal from the Reading Assignment
2 = Element developed in the Reading Assignment
3 = Element which you will recognize through its use in common words or as discussed under Familiar Elements
4 = Element used in Medical Terms Used in Description of Diseases

CODE	ELEMENT	AUDIONYM	MEANING
4	con		together
4	contin		to hold, to contain
0	contra	contractor	against, counter
2	contra		"opposite to," "against"
0	cor	core	heart
2	cord, cor		pertaining to the heart
0	corne	corn	horny, hornlike
2	corne		cornea of the eye
0	cost	coaster	rib
2	counter		"against," "opposite to"
0	crani	crane	skull
4	cret		grow
0	crine	cry'n	to secrete
0	cryo	cry	cold
0	cut	cut	skin
0	cyan	sign	blue
0	cyst	sister	sac containing fluid, bladder
0	cyt	sight	cell
0	dacry	daiquiri	tear
0	dactyl	duck tail	finger, toe
0	dendr	den door	tree, branching (as in nervous system)
0	dent	dentist	teeth
2	derm		skin
0	dermat	doormat	skin
0	desis	thesis	binding, fixation
0	di	dye	twice, double, twofold
0	dia	diet pill	through, across, apart
0	digit	dig it	finger, toe
4	dips		thirst
0	dis	discus	apart, asunder, away, opposite of
3	dist		far
0	dors	doors	back
2	dors		back as landmark, back side
0	duct	duck	tube, channel, canal, lead, draw
0	duodeno		duodenum
4	duplic		double, twofold
0	dura	door	hard
0	dyn	dinner	pain
2	dyn, odyn		pain

ALPHABETICAL LIST OF ELEMENTS, AUDIONYMS (Where Applicable) AND MEANINGS

Description of Code

0 = One of the 350 elements taught in this course
1 = Word terminal from the Reading Assignment
2 = Element developed in the Reading Assignment
3 = Element which you will recognize through its use in common words or as discussed under Familiar Elements
4 = Element used in Medical Terms Used in Description of Diseases

CODE	ELEMENT	AUDIONYM	MEANING
0	dynam	dynamite	power
0	dys	dice	bad, out of order
2	dys		out of order, difficult, painful
2	dystrophy		"bad development," "bad nourishment"
1	e		means of, instrument for
0	ectasis	"egged a sis"	expansion
2	ecto		situated on the outside, outside
0	ectomy	exit Tommy	surgical removal of all or part of
0	edema	a demon	swelling (by fluid)
2	edema		"edema of . . .," or as suffix
3	EENT		ear, eye, nose, throat (acronym)
2	em		blood
2	em		variation of en before b, m, or p
2	embry-		early stage of fertilized egg
2	eme		vomit, vomiting
0	emesis	hey Mrs!	vomiting
0	en	hen	in
2	en, em		in, within, inside
1	ence		variation of ance — state or condition, act of
0	encephal	hen sieve fall	brain
0	end	the end	inside, within
2	end, ent		pointing to
2	ent		inside, within, inner
0	enter	enter (sign)	intestines (usually small)
0	ependym	a pendulum	wrapping, a covering
2	ependym		membrane enclosing brain and spinal cord
0	epi	a pea	upon, in addition to
0	erythro	wreath throw	red
1	es		plural ending similar to -s
1	esis		condition or process
4	esis		go, send
2	eso		inner, inward
0	esophag		esophagus
0	esthesia	has the show	sensation, feeling
2	esthesia		consciousness
0	eu	ukulele	good, well, normal, easy
0	eury, eur	urinal	broad, wide, opposite of narrow
0	ex	eggs	out, away from
2	exo		outside, outward, outer

ALPHABETICAL LIST OF ELEMENTS, AUDIONYMS (Where Applicable) AND MEANINGS

Description of Code

0 = One of the 350 elements taught in this course
1 = Word terminal from the Reading Assignment
2 = Element developed in the Reading Assignment
3 = Element which you will recognize through its use in common words or as discussed under Familiar Elements
4 = Element used in Medical Terms Used in Description of Diseases

CODE	ELEMENT	AUDIONYM	MEANING
2	exterior		more to the outside
2	external		perceived outwardly, outward form, appearance
2	extra		outside of, beyond
2	extra, extro		on the outside, beyond, outer (ext. of ex)
0	fac, fic, fect	factory	make, do, cause
2	fac, fici		face, outer surface, form, figure
0	fascia	face	sheet, band
4	fer		carry
3	fibr		fiber, filament
0	fiss, fid	fish	split, cleave
0	fistul	fist	pipe, a narrow passage
4	flacc		flabby
3	flex, flect		bend, turn
1	form		same form, shaped like, resembling
0	furca	fur coat	fork-shaped
4	fus		melt, join
0	gangli	gang	swelling, knotlike mass
4	gangren		a gnawing away, an eating sore
0	gastr	gas truck	stomach
0	gemin	gem	twin, double
0	gen	genesis	original, production
2	gen		bring forth, arise in, the source of
2	gen		word terminal -producer, that which is produced
2	genesis		process or condition leading to production
2	genic, genous		producing, originating, giving rise to
2	genit		reproduction, the organs or reproduction
0	ger, geron	jar	old, old person, old age
2	geront		old age, old person
0	gingiv	gingerbread (man)	gum
4	gli		glue
4	glob		ball
0	glom	glow	ball
0	glosso	glossy	tongue
4	glut		glue
0	glyco, gluco	glide coal	sweet, sugar
0	grad	graduate	walk, take steps
2	grad		stage in a process
0	gram	graham cracker	record, write
0	gran	grandma	grain, particle

ALPHABETICAL LIST OF ELEMENTS, AUDIONYMS (Where Applicable) AND MEANINGS

Description of Code

0 = One of the 350 elements taught in this course
1 = Word terminal from the Reading Assignment
2 = Element developed in the Reading Assignment
3 = Element which you will recognize through its use in common words or as discussed under Familiar Elements
4 = Element used in Medical Terms Used in Description of Diseases

CODE	ELEMENT	AUDIONYM	MEANING
4	granul		little grain, little particle
0	gravid	gravity	pregnant
0	gyn, gynec	gun, gin	female, woman
2	h		dropping when not initial letter of word
4	halit		breath
0	hallux	hall "X"	great toe
2	hard		comparisons of dura, scirrh, scler
0	helio	heel	sun, light
0	hem(at)	hem	blood
2	hemi		part of
0	hemi	hemisphere	half
0	hepat	he pat	liver
4	hern		intestine, entrails
4	hesion		a sticking
0	heter, (eter)	header	other, different from, opposite
2	hetero		other, different from, opposite
0	histo	his toe	tissue
0	hom, homo	home	same, like, the same as, equal, resembling
2	homo		man, humankind
2	homeo		like, the same as, equal, resembling
0	hormone	harmonize	excite or set in motion
0	hydro	hydrant	water
0	hyper	high purr	above, more than normal
2	hyper		excessive, more than normal
2	hypertrophy		overdevelopment
0	hypno	hypnotist	sleep
0	hypo	hippo	under, beneath, deficient
2	hypo		less than normal, below in space
0	hyster	his stir	uterus, womb
1	ia		disease, unhealthy state or condition
0	iasis	oasis	condition, formation of, presence of
2	iasis		disease process, result of disease
2	iatr		heal, treat, cure
1	ic		pertaining to
1	ical		pertaining to
1	ician		of, belonging to, person who
1	ics		body of facts, knowledge, matters etc.
1	ics, ology		meaning — ics vs ology
1	id		pertaining to, "being"

ALPHABETICAL LIST OF ELEMENTS, AUDIONYMS (Where Applicable) AND MEANINGS

Description of Code

0 = One of the 350 elements taught in this course
1 = Word terminal from the Reading Assignment
2 = Element developed in the Reading Assignment
3 = Element which you will recognize through its use in common words or as discussed under Familiar Elements
4 = Element used in Medical Terms Used in Description of Diseases

CODE	ELEMENT	AUDIONYM	MEANING
1	ide		chemical compound naming
0	ile		ileum
0	ili		ilium
1	in		organic compound ending
3	in, il, im, ir		in, within, inward, toward, into
3	in, il, im, ir		not
0	infer	inn, fur	under, below
3	infero		below and, on the outside
0	infra	infra red oven	beneath
2	integument		skin
0	inter	interpreter	between
3	inter		between, among, in the midst
3	interior		something that is within, more to the inside
3	intern		between (variation of inter)
3	internal		existing or situated within something
0	intra	introduce	within
2	intra		within, during, between layers, underneath
2	intro		in, into, inward, within
1	ion		action, condition resulting from action
1	ior		"comparative," same as English -er
1	ior		roughly meaning "more toward"
0	iris	I race	rainbow (eye membrane)
1	is		noun ending, add to root to form name
0	iso	I sew	equal
1	ist		one who, practices, does, concerned with
1	ition		same as -ation, process, action, condition
0	itis	I test	inflammation
1	ity		condition, character
1	ium		noun end, place, region, lining, covering
1	ive		of, relating to, having nature or quality of
1	ization		action or process, -ize + -ation
0	kerat	carrot	horny, horny tissue
2	kerat		cornea of the eye
2	kin, cin		to move
2	kine		general relationship to movement
2	kinet		movable

ALPHABETICAL LIST OF ELEMENTS, AUDIONYMS (Where Applicable) AND MEANINGS

Description of Code

0 = One of the 350 elements taught in this course
1 = Word terminal from the Reading Assignment
2 = Element developed in the Reading Assignment
3 = Element which you will recognize through its use in common words or as discussed under Familiar Elements
4 = Element used in Medical Terms Used in Description of Diseases

CODE	ELEMENT	AUDIONYM	MEANING
0	labi	lab	lip
0	lacrim	lake rim	tear
0	lact	lacquer	milk
0	lal	lolly (pop)	speech
0	lapar	lap	abdominal wall
2	lapar		lower back and sides
4	lapse		fall, falling
0	laryng		larynx
4	lat		wide
0	later	ladder	side
0	leio	lei	smooth
0	lept	leopard	slender, thin, delicate (literally "peeled")
4	les		injure, hurt, wound
4	let		little, small
0	leuk	Look (magazine)	white
0	lien	line (clothes)	spleen
0	lig		ligament
2	lig		tie, bind
2	lig, ligat		to bind, tie
4	lim		hunger
0	lingua	language	tongue
0	lip	lip	fat
0	lith	lather	stone
0	lobo	low bow	section
3	loc		place
0	lumbo	lumber	loins
1	ly		in a manner, way, by way of, toward
0	lymph	limp	watery fluid, major fluid of body
0	lysis	license	loosening, destruction, set free
0	macro	macaroni	large
0	macul	Mack (truck)	spot (or stain)
0	mal	mall	bad
2	mal		abnormal, faulty, poor (inadequate, insufficient)
0	malacia	my late show (TV)	soft condition
0	malign	my leg	bad, harmful
0	mamm	mammal	breast
0	mani	maniac	madness, mental disturbance
2	manu		hand
0	mast	mast	breast

ALPHABETICAL LIST OF ELEMENTS, AUDIONYMS (Where Applicable) AND MEANINGS

Description of Code

0 = One of the 350 elements taught in this course
1 = Word terminal from the Reading Assignment
2 = Element developed in the Reading Assignment
3 = Element which you will recognize through its use in common words or as discussed under Familiar Elements
4 = Element used in Medical Terms Used in Description of Diseases

CODE	ELEMENT	AUDIONYM	MEANING
2	mat		variation for roots ending in m
0	maxill	makes hill	upper jawbone
0	mechano	mechanic	machine
0	med	meat	middle
4	medull		marrow, pith
0	megal	my gal	enlarged
0	melan	melon	black
0	mening	manage	membrane
0	ment	mint	mind
2	mes		middle, intermediate
0	meta	metal cabinet	beyond, change, transformation, after
0	metabole	met a bull	change
0	metr	meter	uterus
0	mi	mice	less
0	micr	microphone	small
2	mio, meio		less, smaller
3	mono		one, alone, single, limited to one part
0	morph	mower roof	form, shape, finger
4	motil		movement
4	motility		movement
3	multi		many, much, more than one
3	muscul		muscle
0	my	my eye	muscle
0	myco	my comb	fungus
0	myel	mile	marrow (spinal cord)
0	myring	my ring	eardrum
3	narc, narcot		numbness, stupor, apathy
3	nas		nose
0	necr	neck	dead
0	neo	kneel	new
0	nephr	nephew	kidney
1	ness		state, quality, instance of being
0	neuro	Nero	nerve or nervous system
2	nex		join
4	nomaly		distributed
4	non		not
0	ocul	a "kool"	eye
2	ocul		relationship to the eye, landmark use
0	odont	oh don't	tooth
0	oid	void	like, resembling

ALPHABETICAL LIST OF ELEMENTS, AUDIONYMS (Where Applicable) AND MEANINGS

Description of Code

0 = One of the 350 elements taught in this course
1 = Word terminal from the Reading Assignment
2 = Element developed in the Reading Assignment
3 = Element which you will recognize through its use in common words or as discussed under Familiar Elements
4 = Element used in Medical Terms Used in Description of Diseases

CODE	ELEMENT	AUDIONYM	MEANING
0	olfact	oil factory	smell, odor, to smell
0	ologist	hollow chest	a specialist in the study of
0	ology	hollow cheese	study of
0	oma	Oh Ma!	tumor
2	oma		swelling, mass of new tissue growth
2	omat		tumor
0	oment	"O" men	covering (of internal abdominal organs)
0	onco	uncle	tumor, mass, or swelling
0	onych	onyx	nail, claw
2	onych		fingernail, toenail
2	oo		egg or ovum
0	oophor	over	ovary
4	opac		dark, shaded
0	ophthalm, opt	up thumb	eye
2	ophthalm		relationship to the eye
2	opia		suffix denotes condition of vision, sight
2	opt		seeing, vision, light
2	opt		visible, relationship to vision or sight
0	or	oar	mouth
1	or		action, result, performer, functional
1	or		person or thing that performs, functions
0	orchi	orchid	testis
2	orchi		male reproductive gland
4	orexia		desire, appetite
0	orth	Orthodox church	straight, correct, normal
0	osis	OH Sis!	condition, any condition
0	osmo	I smoke	odor
2	oss		bone
2	osse		bone
2	ossi		bone
0	ost	ostrich	bone
2	oste		bone
0	ostomy	Oh stop Tommy!	to create an opening
2	otic, otid		ear as landmark, situated in ear area
0	oto	"O" toe	ear
0	otomy	Oh Tommy!	cut into, incision into
1	ous		full of, abounding in, having
2	ov-		egg, ovar as egg container
0	ovar	over	egg (the female reproductive gland)
0	ovario		ovary

ALPHABETICAL LIST OF ELEMENTS, AUDIONYMS (Where Applicable) AND MEANINGS

Description of Code

0 = One of the 350 elements taught in this course
1 = Word terminal from the Reading Assignment
2 = Element developed in the Reading Assignment
3 = Element which you will recognize through its use in common words or as discussed under Familiar Elements
4 = Element used in Medical Terms Used in Description of Diseases

CODE	ELEMENT	AUDIONYM	MEANING
0	pachy	pack	thick
4	pact		press
3	palat		palate, the roof of the mouth
0	palpebr	pile of people	eyelid
0	pan	pan	all
2	pant		variation of pan, all, completely, the whole
4	papill		nipple
0	para	parachute	beside, beyond
2	para		beyond, wrong, faculty, disordered
0	pariet	parrot	wall
0	part	part	labor, bring forth
2	part		to separate from
0	path	path	disease
0	pect, pector	pecked	chest, breast, thorax
2	ped		foot or child
2	pelv		pelvis, ring of bones in hip area
0	pelvis		pelvis
0	penia	pen	decrease
0	peps, pept	pepsi	digest
0	per	purr	throughout, through, thoroughly, excessively
0	peri	pear	about, around
2	peri		peri, o, . . . ium, peri, o, . . . eum, tissue
2	peri		surrounding, enclosing, covering
4	petechiae		small spots
0	pexy	pecks egg	suspension fixation
2	pexy		surgical act of fastening or securing
0	phage	page	to eat
2	phage		swallowing
0	phak	vacuum cleaner	lens
0	pharmac	farm axe	drug
0	pharyng		pharynx
0	phleb	flip	vein
0	phob	foe	fear
0	phon	phone	voice, sound
2	phon		speech or body sounds
2	phor		carrier
0	phot	photo	light
0	phrag, phrax	fur rag	fence, to fence in, wall off, block up
0	phren	friend	mind
2	phren		diaphragm

215

ALPHABETICAL LIST OF ELEMENTS, AUDIONYMS (Where Applicable) AND MEANINGS

Description of Code

0 = One of the 350 elements taught in this course
1 = Word terminal from the Reading Assignment
2 = Element developed in the Reading Assignment
3 = Element which you will recognize through its use in common words or as discussed under Familiar Elements
4 = Element used in Medical Terms Used in Description of Diseases

CODE	ELEMENT	AUDIONYM	MEANING
0	physio	physics	nature
2	physio		the body (frequently as opposed to the mind)
4	pica		magpie (omniverous eater)
0	pilo	pile on	hair
0	plak	plaque	plate
2	plak		a patch of eruption
2	plak, plax		flat or board plate, a patch of eruptio
0	plasia	play show	development or growth
0	plast	plastic (cement)	surgical repair, plastic repair
2	plast		renewal, reforming reconstruction
0	platy	plate	flat, broad
0	plegia	pledge	paralysis
2	plegia		loss of power
0	pleur	pliers	pleura (membrane), rib, side
2	pleura		membrane covering the chest cavity
0	plexus	plexiglass	braid, an inter weaving or network
2	pne		air or breathing
2	pnea		breathing
0	pneum	name	lung, air
2	pneum, pneumat		relationship to air or respiration
2	pneumon		relationship to lungs
0	pod	pod	foot
0	poly	polish	much, many
0	post	post office	after, behind
0	poster	poster	back part, behind, rear
0	pre	pray	in front of, before
0	pro		in front of, before
0	proct	Procter & Gamble	anus
2	proct		designating rectum, anal canal
0	proli	parolee	offspring
0	proxim	peroxide	nearest, near
0	pseud	false teeth	false, imaginary, spurious
0	psycho	cycle	mind
0	ptosis	toe Sis	falling, drooping
4	pty		saliva, spittle
0	ptyal	tile	saliva (pretaining to)
0	puer	pure (gold)	child
0	pulmon, pulmo	pull moon	lung
2	pulmon		lung as landmark
0	pyle, pyloro	pie	gate

216

ALPHABETICAL LIST OF ELEMENTS, AUDIONYMS (Where Applicable) AND MEANINGS

Description of Code

0 = One of the 350 elements taught in this course
1 = Word terminal from the Reading Assignment
2 = Element developed in the Reading Assignment
3 = Element which you will recognize through its use in common words or as discussed under Familiar Elements
4 = Element used in Medical Terms Used in Description of Diseases

CODE	ELEMENT	AUDIONYM	MEANING
2	plyor		"gatekeeper"
0	rachi	rake	spinal column
0	radi	radio	ray
0	radic	radish	root
0	ramus	ram	branch
3	re		back, back again, contrary, opposite
0	ren	rain	kidney
0	retro	retreat	backwards
2	retro		contrary to the usual or natural course
0	rhag, rrhag	raging river	burst forth, break, burst, rupture
2	rhagad		a split, crack, fissure
2	rrhagia		heavy bleeding
0	rhaphy	raffle	suture, suturing
0	rhe, rrhe	reed instrument	flow, to flow
0	rhexis	wrecks	break, burst
2	rhexis		rupture, forcible tearing apart
0	rhin	rhinoceros	nose
2	rrh		rrh vs rh in elements
2	rrhex		to break, burst, rupture
2	ruct		belch
0	rug	rug	wrinkle, fold, crease
4	rupt		break
0	sacro		sacrum
0	salpingo	Sally bingo	tube
2	salpingo		esp. the uterus
0	sarc	shark	flesh
0	schiz	skis	to split, cleave
0	scirr	skirt	hard
2	scirrh, scirr		variation of scirr, hard cancerous tumor
0	sclera	scholar	hard
0	scol, scoli	school	curved, twisted, crooked
2	scolec		worm-shaped
0	scop	scope	look, observe
4	secret		set apart, hidden
3	sect		a cut or division, to cut or divide
0	sedat	seated	quiet, calm
0	semen	seaman	seed
0	semi	semi colon	half
2	semi		partially
4	sen		old

ALPHABETICAL LIST OF ELEMENTS, AUDIONYMS (Where Applicable) AND MEANINGS

Description of Code

0 = One of the 350 elements taught in this course
1 = Word terminal from the Reading Assignment
2 = Element developed in the Reading Assignment
3 = Element which you will recognize through its use in common words or as discussed under Familiar Elements
4 = Element used in Medical Terms Used in Description of Diseases

CODE	ELEMENT	AUDIONYM	MEANING
0	sept	sipped	wall, fence
2	sept		dividing wall or membrane
4	sin		curve, fold, bend
0	sinus	sign us	hollow space
3	skelet		skeleton, the bony framework of the body
0	somato	sew my toe	body
0	somni	"saw my knee"	sleep
0	spas	space	pull, draw
0	spasm	spaceman	involuntary contractions
0	sphenic	sphinx	wedge, wedge-shaped
0	spiro	sparrow	coil
2	spiro		winding, twisting
0	splanchn(o)	"S" plank	internal organs, viscera
0	splen		spleen
0	spondyl	spun doll	spinal column or vertebra
0	squam	squaw	scale
0	sta, stas, ste	stand	stand, to cause to stand, set, fix
0	steno	stenographer	narrow, contracted
2	stenosis		constriction of a passage in the body
2	steth		chest
2	sthen		strength, strong
4	stip		press
2	stom, stomy		new opening = a mouth or opening
0	stoma	stone	mouth or opening
4	strangul		a squeezing, choking
0	strept	stripped	twist
0	strict	strict	a draw tight, narrowing
0	sub	submarine	under, beneath, below
2	sub		less than
2	super		above, relation to supra
3	super		over, above, higher inquantity or quality
0	supra	soup	above, over
0	syn, sym	cymbals	together
0	tarso	tar	ankle region, instep
0	tarso		framework of the upper eyelid
2	tas, tend, tens		to stretch
0	tegument	tag you men	covering or skin
2	tein (tan, ten)		to stretch
2	tele		distant, far away
2	ten		stretch, a stretcher, stretching (extend)

ALPHABETICAL LIST OF ELEMENTS, AUDIONYMS (Where Applicable) AND MEANINGS

Description of Code

0 = One of the 350 elements taught in this course
1 = Word terminal from the Reading Assignment
2 = Element developed in the Reading Assignment
3 = Element which you will recognize through its use in common words or as discussed under Familiar Elements
4 = Element used in Medical Terms Used in Description of Diseases

CODE	ELEMENT	AUDIONYM	MEANING
0	tens	tents	stretch
4	terat		monster, monstrous
2	tetan		stretched, spasm
0	thalam	the lamb	inner chamber
0	thel	the "L"	nipple
0	therap		therapy
0	therm	thermomenter	heat
0	thorac	throw rock	chest
0	thromb	trombone	lump, clot
0	thyro		thyroid
1	tic		pertaining to
0	ton	ton	stretching, a stretching, tension
2	top		place, locality, localized
0	tope	top	place
3	tors, tort		twist, turn
3	tox		poison
2	trache		windpipe
0	trachel	tray coal	neck or necklike structure
4	tract		draw
0	trans	trains	through, across, beyond
2	trauma		shock, stress, injury
0	traumat	laundromat	wound, injury
4	tres		hole, opening
0	tri		three
2	tri		involving three, triply, third
0	trich	trick	hair
0	trip	trip	rub, friction
2	trip		friction
0	trophy	trophy	development, growth
2	trophy		nutrition, nourishment
4	trus		thrust, push
4	tum		swell
0	tumor	two more	swelling
0	turbin	turban	shaped like a top
0	tympan	tin fan	eardrum or its enclosure
1	ular		pertaining to
1	ular		pertaining to a small version
1	ule		small, little
4	ul		small
3	ultra		beyond, excessive

ALPHABETICAL LIST OF ELEMENTS, AUDIONYMS (Where Applicable) AND MEANINGS

Description of Code

0 = One of the 350 elements taught in this course
1 = Word terminal from the Reading Assignment
2 = Element developed in the Reading Assignment
3 = Element which you will recognize through its use in common words or as discussed under Familiar Elements
4 = Element used in Medical Terms Used in Description of Diseases

CODE	ELEMENT	AUDIONYM	MEANING
1	um		noun ending, add to root to form name
0	umbilic	a bill lick	navel
1	ure		result of action, means of action, device
0	ureter		ureter
0	urethra		urethra
1	us		noun ending, name forming from root
0	utero		uterus
0	vaso	vase	vessel
0	vena		vein
0	ventr	vent	front, belly, abdomen, cavity
2	vermi		worm, wormlike
0	vert	vertebrae	turn
3	vertebr-		vertebra, bones of the spinal column
0	vesic	vest sick	bladder
0	vestibule	vest bull	entrance
2	vestibule		space or cavity at entrance to a canal
0	viscero	vice row	organ
2	viscero		internal organ, internal organs
0	volv	valve	to roll, turn, roll over, a turning
2	volut		a turning or rolling motion
0	vulse	false	twitch or pull
0	xer	zero	dry
1	y		act or result of act, condition, quality

Name: _____ Date: _____

The Dean Vaughn Learning System
MEDICAL TERMINOLOGY

100% AWARD
FINAL TEST

Number correct: _____

Possible Score: _____ *350* _____

Percent Correct: _____ %

Important:

Clearly print the meaning of each element in the blank where indicated. A space has been provided for you to also include its audionym as an aid in recalling the meaning. This step is optional. You will be tested on the meanings of the elements only.

MEDICAL TERMINOLOGY FINAL TEST

ELEMENT	AUDIONYM	MEANING
1. gastr-		
2. cardi-		
3. megal-		
4. -itis		
5. dermat-		
6. plast-		
7. cerebr-		
8. path-		
9. -ectomy		
10. enter-		
11. -osis		
12. -otomy		
13. aden-		
14. angi-		
15. -oma		
16. nephr-		
17. hepat-		
18. arthr-		
19. blephar-		
20. -ologist		
21. rhin-		
22. gingiv-		
23. -malacia		
24. -ology		
25. spasm		

MEDICAL TERMINOLOGY FINAL TEST

ELEMENT	AUDIONYM	MEANING
26. -algia	-------------------------	_____
27. crani-	-------------------------	_____
28. end-	-------------------------	_____
29. hemi-	-------------------------	_____
30. oid-	-------------------------	_____
31. hyper-	-------------------------	_____
32. cyst	-------------------------	_____
33. chole-	-------------------------	_____
34. hypo-	-------------------------	_____
35. -scop-	-------------------------	_____
36. hyster-	-------------------------	_____
37. -ostomy	-------------------------	_____
38. para-	-------------------------	_____
39. -lysis	-------------------------	_____
40. cervic-	-------------------------	_____
41. chondr-	-------------------------	_____
42. cyan-	-------------------------	_____
43. hem(at)-	-------------------------	_____
44. ost-	-------------------------	_____
45. psycho-	-------------------------	_____
46. lip-	-------------------------	_____
47. my-	-------------------------	_____
48. lith-	-------------------------	_____
49. ophthalm- opt-	-------------------------	_____
50. proct-	-------------------------	_____

MEDICAL TERMINOLOGY FINAL TEST

ELEMENT	AUDIONYM	MEANING
51. cost-		
52. -gram		
53. acro-		
54. rhexis		
55. carcin-		
56. -penia		
57. gen-		
58. burso-		
59. retr(o)-		
60. trip-		
61. strept-		
62. -desis		
63. mani-		
64. glosso-		
65. -trophy		
66. supra-		
67. -ptosis		
68. dyn-		
69. mast-		
70. -rrhaphy		
71. dent-		
72. cephal-		
73. auto-		
74. epi-		
75. hydro-		

MEDICAL TERMINOLOGY FINAL TEST

ELEMENT	AUDIONYM	MEANING
76. lobo-		
77. -emesis		
78. contra-		
79. -iasis		
80. trans-		
81. brady-		
82. -ectasis		
83. cyt-		
84. odont-		
85. leuk-		
86. -esthesia		
87. cantho-		
88. steno-		
89. cheil-		
90. -cele		
91. benign		
92. semen		
93. celio-		
94. erythro-		
95. vaso-		
96. melan-		
97. cauda-		
98. lingua-		
99. myring-		
100. spondyl-		

MEDICAL TERMINOLOGY FINAL TEST

ELEMENT	AUDIONYM	MEANING
101. ovar-		
102. -centesis		
103. oto-		
104. bili-		
105. squam-		
106. mening-		
107. cec-		
108. macul-		
109. -pexy		
110. onco-		
111. or-		
112. sub-		
113. spiro-		
114. lacrim-		
115. viscero-		
116. lact-		
117. onych-		
118. thorac-		
119. pyle- pyloro-		
120. vesic-		
121. sphenic-		
122. myel-		
123. anti-		
124. myco-		
125. hallux-		

NAME ———————————————————— DATE ————————

MEDICAL TERMINOLOGY FINAL TEST

ELEMENT	AUDIONYM	MEANING
126. physio-		
127. bucco-		
128. palpebr-		
129. plasia-		
130. rug-		
131. aur-		
132. acousti-		
133. colpo-		
134. phon-		
135. leio-		
136. cor		
137. ren-		
138. orchi-		
139. encephal-		
140. thalam-		
141. plexus		
142. cilia		
143. dendr-		
144. phleb-		
145. pilo-		
146. histo-		
147. stoma-		
148. tympan-		
149. umbilic-		
150. salpingo-		

227

MEDICAL TERMINOLOGY FINAL TEST

ELEMENT	AUDIONYM	MEANING
151. helio-		
152. astr-		
153. -asthenia		
154. fascia		
155. iso-		
156. tarso-		
157. -tope		
158. pod-		
159. malign-		
160. adnexa-		
161. ocul-		
162. lapar-		
163. dacry-		
164. ment-		
165. part-		
166. scler(a)-		
167. somato-		
168. trachel-		
169. sinus		
170. hypno-		
171. sept-		
172. scirr(h)-		
173. antr-		
174. -crine		
175. dura		

MEDICAL TERMINOLOGY FINAL TEST

ELEMENT	AUDIONYM	MEANING
176. pneum-		
177. phage		
178. phren-		
179. corne-		
180. plak-		
181. iris		
182. kerat-		
183. pulmon-		
184. ptyal-		
185. alveol-		
186. oophor-		
187. oment-		
188. sedat-		
189. furca-		
190. radic-		
191. radi-		
192. fistul-		
193. edema-		
194. dactyl-		
195. metabol(e)-		
196. pariet-		
197. ependym-		
198. gravid		
199. aer-		
200. glyco-		

MEDICAL TERMINOLOGY FINAL TEST

ELEMENT	AUDIONYM	MEANING
201. tarso-		
202. cheir- chir-		
203. calc-		
204. cine-		
205. digit		
206. dors-		
207. gangli-		
208. gemin-		
209. grad-		
210. gran-		
211. labi-		
212. micr-		
213. peps- pept-		
214. pleur-		
215. mamm-		
216. colla-		
217. later-		
218. rachi-		
219. phob-		
220. phot-		
221. dys-		
222. cut-		
223. en-		
224. peri-		

MEDICAL TERMINOLOGY FINAL TEST

ELEMENT	AUDIONYM	MEANING
225. pro-		
226. mechano-		
227. dynam-		
228. osmo-		
229. traumat-		
230. trich-		
231. maxill-		
232. an-, a-		
233. phak-		
234. pre-		
235. strict-		
236. turbin-		
237. ameb-		
238. semi-		
239. neo-		
240. hormone		
241. therm-		
242. syn- or sym-		
243. vuls(e)-		
244. post		
245. metr-		
246. tegument		
247. pan-		
248. poly-		
249. ramus		

MEDICAL TERMINOLOGY FINAL TEST

ELEMENT	AUDIONYM	MEANING
250. neuro-		
251. thromb-		
252. ab-		
253. -plegia		
254. ante-		
255. thel-		
256. ex-		
257. lien-		
258. tumor		
259. vestibule		
260. puer-		
261. sarc-		
262. proli-		
263. macro-		
264. lal-		
265. intra-		
266. inter-		
267. infra-		
268. cryo-		
269. mal-		
270. glom-		
271. tens-		
272. spas-		
273. somni-		
274. pharmac-		
275. lumbo-		

MEDICAL TERMINOLOGY FINAL TEST

ELEMENT	MEANING
276. arter-	_____
277. appendic-	_____
278. thyro-	_____
279. splen-	_____
280. ovario-	_____
281. adreno-	_____
282. basi-	_____
283. pelvis	_____
284. vena-	_____
285. urethra	_____
286. utero-	_____
287. sacro-	_____
288. pharyng-	_____
289. duodeno-	_____
290. ureter	_____
291. laryng-	_____
292. bronch-	_____
293. col-	_____
294. esophag-	_____
295. bi-	_____
296. tri-	_____
297. ile-	_____
298. ili-	_____
299. lig-	_____
300. therap-	_____

MEDICAL TERMINOLOGY FINAL TEST

ELEMENT	AUDIONYM	MEANING
301. xer-		
302. sta-		
303. proxim-		
304. morph-		
305. necr-		
306. dia-		
307. di-		
308. fac-		
309. pect-		
310. lymph-		
311. ton-		
312. -rrhe		
313. heter-		
314. per-		
315. volv-		
316. lept-		
317. blast-		
318. meta-		
319. apo-		
320. mi-		
321. scol-		
322. eury-		
323. dis-		
324. med-		
325. -rrhag		

MEDICAL TERMINOLOGY FINAL TEST

ELEMENT	AUDIONYM	MEANING
326. splanchn-		
327. ger-		
328. capit-		
329. ventr-		
330. cau-		
331. vert-		
332. clas-		
333. eu-		
334. fiss-		
335. ambi-		
336. brachy-		
337. amphi-		
338. duct-		
339. poster-		
340. gyn-		
341. hom-		
342. cata-		
343. schiz-		
344. olfact-		
345. pseud-		
346. infer-		
347. pachy-		
348. phrag-		
349. platy-		
350. orth-		